Growing Old, Going Cold

GROWING

OLD,

GOING

COLD

*Notes on Swimming,
Aging, and Finishing Last*

KATHLEEN MCDONNELL

Second Story Press

Library and Archives Canada Cataloguing in Publication

Title: Growing old, going cold : notes on swimming, aging, and
   finishing last / Kathleen McDonnell.
Names: McDonnell, Kathleen, 1947- author.
Identifiers: Canadiana (print) 20210302100 | Canadiana (ebook)
   20210302232 | ISBN 9781772602555 (softcover) | ISBN
   9781772602562 (EPUB)
Subjects: LCSH: McDonnell, Kathleen, 1947- | LCSH: Swimmers—
   Ontario—Biography. | LCSH: Swimming—Ontario, Lake
   (N.Y. and Ont.) | LCGFT: Autobiographies.
Classification: LCC GV838.M33 A3 2022 | DDC 797.2/1092—dc23

Cover by Natalie Olsen

Cover photo: Sunset Swim by Emily Jean Thomas / Stocksy

Editor: Talin Vartanian

Printed and bound in Canada

*Second Story Press gratefully acknowledges the support of the
Ontario Arts Council and the Canada Council for the Arts for our
publishing program. We acknowledge the financial support of the
Government of Canada through the Canada Book Fund.*

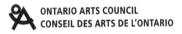

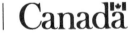

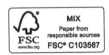

Published by
Second Story Press
20 Maud Street, Suite 401
Toronto, Ontario, Canada
M5V 2M5
www.secondstorypress.ca

For Michael Terence McDonnell, 1944-1981

TABLE OF CONTENTS

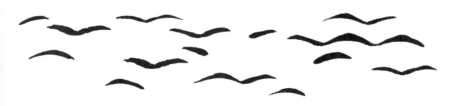

Dip [her] in the river who loves water

FROM *PROVERBS OF HELL* BY WILLIAM BLAKE

PROLOGUE

Growing Old:
Who, me?

ON THE AFTERNOON of September 2, 2017, I walked into Lake Ontario.

Nothing remarkable about that. Over the past three decades I've probably gone into the water off Ward's Island more than a thousand times. This was just another day at the beach, and yet it was something more than that. I was embarking on a Challenge.

Like many amateur athletes, swimmers love to set themselves capital-C Challenges, sometimes extreme ones, like swimming the English Channel or crossing one of the Great Lakes. But mostly they're more ordinary, everyday challenges, like entering a race or setting a self-imposed goal, and the satisfaction and bragging rights that come with reaching it. As this book will make clear, I am not one of those high-achieving types, constantly driving myself to go faster-farther-bigger. But in the fall of 2017, I was facing a huge life transition, one I wasn't entirely happy about. I needed to do something to mark it.

I resolved to swim 70 kilometers between September 2 and October 24, 2017, the day I would turn seventy years of age.

It wasn't going to be a particularly daunting task. I had fifty-two days to achieve my goal, which worked out to a pace of less than 1.5 kilometers (almost a mile) a day. I swim that much as a matter of routine during the summer months; but this was early autumn, and I figured I'd need a head start before Lake Ontario began to cool down. By late October, the temp would have dropped to 10–12 C (50–53.6 F). I'd keep swimming, of course, but I'd have to cut down my time in the water.

Fall has always been my favorite season for swimming. There are fewer people on the beach, and the cooler water suits me just fine. Working toward an objective has always helped me kickstart, mentally and physically, but as the kilometers added up and I got closer and closer to the end point, I found an ambivalence, even a kind of melancholy, creeping into my mood. Forty may be the new thirty, sixty the new fifty. But seventy? Seventy isn't the "new" anything. It's just *old*. Even the day I swam the last kilometer, I didn't feel triumphant the way I had on completing my 365-day swim the year before. I wasn't at all sure that turning seventy was something to celebrate.

That ambivalence continued right through the writing of this book, especially as I struggled to come up with a title. I thought it should have the word "cold" in it, but the ones that kept popping into my head all used "old." I thought about toning it down and using "older" instead, which would mean tossing aside a very nice rhyme. Then I thought I should go in an entirely different direction. How about "crone," the word that feminists reclaimed as a positive term for an older woman back in the seventies? It never really caught on, and the only synonym that wasn't unabashedly negative was the archaic term "beldam." Ah, no. I consulted web articles on best book titles and the advice I gleaned boiled down to this: "The title should explain clearly what the book is about." Thanks a lot.

I've lived most of my life looking younger than my age. I love the shock on people's faces when I tell them how old I am. "No! You can't be!" I'm proud of the many times I've stumped the guy at the "Guess Your Age" booth at the Canadian National Exhibition. What makes it doubly strange for me is I've always found it hard to think of myself as anything but "younger than." When you come from a large family and you're the eighth of nine children, you spend the rest of your life *feeling* younger than everyone around you. Now it's the opposite. I'm older than most people I know.

Over the past decade, I grew reluctant to tell people how old I was. Being coy, even secretive, about one's age—how un-feminist is that? But we all know that getting old is tough on women. There's the double standard: An older man is "distinguished," an older woman is…a bit pathetic? If she's noticed at all. Numerous commentators have noted the ways in which women become, in essence, invisible as they age. I finally came to accept that there was no getting around the reality of my situation; best to embrace it. So there it is, right on the cover of this book: I'm officially, indisputably old.

So much for the invisibility of the older woman.

Don't get me wrong. This book is not a lament for my aging self or anyone else's. I've discovered a secret formula. It's not quite the fountain of youth, but it's the greatest anti-aging potion ever discovered: cold water. It amazes me that, as I move into old age, I've finally found something I can do that few other people can. I'm not really brave or tough, though I enjoy that people think I am. Cold-water swimming is the only physical activity that I am, by some miracle, innately good at. It has made my life immeasurably better.

There are people who are indifferent to water. There are people who hate getting wet. And there are people like me who can't see a body of water without thinking about jumping into it. Is it astrological? My sign is Scorpio, and my chart is mostly water. I love being in water. I can't live without it. In an earlier book I wrote, about an eighteenth-century feral child, I described how she was forbidden to swim as part of a campaign to "civilize" her and how this felt, to me, like "a fate worse than death." As melodramatic as that sounds, it's true.

In more ways than I can count, swimming has come to define my life. As I become more acutely aware that my time on this planet—consisting mostly of water—is diminishing, it's truer than ever.

CHAPTER 1

Dancing about Architecture:
Writing about swimming

"WRITING ABOUT MUSIC is like dancing about architecture." Maybe you've heard this quote before or seen it floating around the Internet, where it's variously attributed to Frank Zappa, Thelonius Monk, David Byrne... the list goes on. The web is rife with phony quotes and false attributions that people naively pass around as nuggets of wisdom from celebrities. I've fallen for the odd one myself (though I'm too proud to fill in the details). At least I'm savvy enough to know that Albert Einstein never said, "Evil is the result of what happens when man does not have God's love present in his heart." In a speech in 2017, then-US President Donald Trump quoted Abraham Lincoln to the effect of "It's not the years in your life that count, it's the life in your years." What a wit, that Abe. I wonder which of Trump's speechwriters dug that up. Another one attributed to Lincoln is a near-universal favorite of phony-quote connoisseurs: "The problem with Internet quotes is that you cannot always depend on their accuracy" sometimes dumbed down to "Don't believe everything you read on the Internet."

There is evidence the architecture quote can, in fact, be traced to an interview with the actor Martin Mull in a 1979 pop music magazine. Mull's quip was picked up and quoted by musician Elvis Costello in a 1983 interview. Whoever came up with it, I think it's persisted because it sums up the ineffability of the experience of music. A phrase like "you had to be there" expresses much the same thing, the inadequacy of words to substitute for direct experience.

I'm a writer and a swimmer. I've engaged in both activities for many decades, but I've always kept the two entirely separate. Write about swimming? Why? What would I say? What was there *to* say about water and the act of moving through it? It seemed to me that it was a case of *you have to be there*, that writing about swimming would be too removed from the immediacy, the tactility, the floating state of mind. Kind of like, yes, dancing about architecture. My attitude changed when I embarked on a plan to swim outdoors every day for an entire year, an undertaking that cried out to be documented. At the end of that year of journaling, I realized I did have something to say about swimming—a lot more than I'd realized. I also discovered I wasn't alone. It turns out there's a whole genre of memoirs about swimming, with its own catchphrase: swimoirs!

In recent years, swimming memoirs have become the

new self-help books. A striking number of them are by women, and many have a healing theme: from addiction (Amy Liptrot's *The Outrun*); to trauma and depression (*I Found My Tribe*, by Ruth Fitzmaurice); to infertility and the ravages of IVF treatments (*Leap In: A Woman, Some Waves, and the Will to Swim*, by Alexandra Heminsley). Some, like Bonnie Tsui's more recent *Why We Swim*, are a hybrid of memoir and reportage. She interviews a range of swimmers and scientists, even an archaeologist who's studying fourteen-thousand-year-old evidence of swimming during the period known as the Green Sahara (who knew the Sahara used to be green?).

Quite a few Canadians have written swimoirs too. Some have a strong eco-political bent, like *The Big Swim: Coming Ashore in a World Adrift*, by Carrie Saxifrage. In the healing vein is *Turning: A Year in the Water*, in which author Jessica J. Lee recounts how a year of swimming in fifty-two lakes, in and around Berlin, helped her through a marriage breakup. In her 2012 memoir, *Swimming Studies*, Leanne Shapton chronicles and illustrates (with her own artwork) training for the Olympics as a teenager, and how that experience left its mark long after her life as a competitive swimmer ended.

But there are only so many ways you can describe arriving at a lake or seashore, locking up your bike, the surroundings, the feel of the water, etc. The reviews tend to be repetitive, and words like "haunting" and "lyrical" turn up often. There's no doubt that swimoirs are having their cultural moment, but we all owe a huge debt to two very different writers, whose pioneering books demonstrated that writing about swimming can be downright illuminating: *Haunts of the Black Masseur: The Swimmer as Hero*, by Charles Sprawson, and Roger Deakin's *Waterlog: A Swimmer's Journey Through Britain*.

Sprawson was the first contemporary writer to focus so intently on the experience of swimming. *Haunts of the Black Masseur* garnered praise on its publication in 1992, and its influence has been significant and enduring. But even the book's most devoted fans readily admit that it's a strange piece of work, starting with the title; a reference to an even stranger Tennessee Williams short story from the late forties. If you're not steeped in British intellectual history, you likely won't get a lot of his offhand literary references. Even more offhand is his account of his own swimming challenge: Lord Byron's legendary swim of the Hellespont, the mile-wide natural strait in northwestern Turkey that forms part of the continental boundary between Europe and Asia, now called the Dardanelles. Unlike other swim memoirists, he disposes of his own remarkable feat in a couple of sentences.

To his credit, Sprawson is much more interested in recounting stories of other swimmers than he is in writing about himself. *Haunts* is packed with fascinating, dramatic, and sometimes bizarre tales of swimming lore from history and literature. Sprawson writes about Matthew Webb, the first person to complete an unassisted swim across the English Channel in 1875, and how his overweening drive to top his own achievements was his undoing. Many warned Webb that his attempt to swim the whirlpool below Niagara Falls in 1883 was impossible, even suicidal. But he had to try. "He dived from the boat and swam away. He was never seen alive again," Sprawson intones, melodramatically.

He's also fascinated with the swimming world's legacy to Hollywood in the thirties and forties, exploring the careers of "aquamusical" star Esther Williams and Olympic swimmer Johnny Weissmuller, who starred in a dozen Tarzan movies. But Sprawson's interests are not all frivolous. He devotes a good deal of space to Australian swimmer Annette Kellermann and her remarkable recovery from childhood paralysis. Born with congenital weakness in her legs, Kellermann "swam her way out of metal braces and into good health." She became part of the international swimming elite, setting a number of distance records, and made three attempts to be the first woman to swim the English Channel—eventually achieved by Gertrude Ederle in 1926. Kellermann was also a feminist trailblazer, rejecting the bulky, modest swimsuits of the early twentieth century to design swimwear that allowed her—and other women—to cut loose in the water.

Sprawson never wrote another book. He died in January 2020 at the age of seventy-eight, before he finished a second book about the Slovenian endurance swimmer Martin Strel (about whom you'll hear more later in this book).

In sharp contrast to Sprawson, Roger Deakins' *Waterlog* is almost exclusively focused on a single swimmer: the author himself. In the nineties, he set out on a year-long journey through the waterways of Britain on a quest to experience life in what he called a feral state: "For the best part of a year, the water would become my natural habitat," he wrote. To Deakins, the act of swimming is "to experience how it was before you were born.... You are in nature...in a far more complete and intense way than on dry land."

The swimmers described in *Haunts of the Black Masseur* are mostly competitive champions. But Deakins's book comes at the subject from a very different, almost unique perspective. I think this is because he isn't primarily a swimmer, he's a *bather*. The Brits traditionally use the word bathing interchangeably with swimming. It's a practice that runs throughout *Waterlog* but won't appear much in this book. (I'm more a bather than a swimmer myself, but having grown up in North America, I can't shake the word's association with bathtubs and getting clean.) Deakins's primary drive is to get *into* the water. He wants to fully *experience* it rather than conquer it, to become part of the water and vice versa. His specialty is distance, rather than speed. Competitive swimmers keep their heads down to maximize speed, but not Deakins. His head is up, looking at his surroundings and the abundant wildlife, especially waterbirds, because he prefers breaststroke. (At one point Deakins is informed by an Australian swimmer that "real men" don't do breaststroke!) He also bathes in rivers, shallow, muddy-bottomed "lodes" in the Fens—bodies of water that conventional, competitive swimmers wouldn't bother with.

Waterlog is also a journey through England's history via its waterways. Deakins swims in every region of the country (or declines to swim, as he did Lord Byron's famous pool in Cambridge, dismayed by its proximity to a superhighway). He explores the specificity of each place by the changes in the landscape and waterways through time, both the recent and distant past. He even entertains an obscure theory that humans may have spent eons as sea-dwellers before moving to dry land: "Perhaps we are more at home in or around water than on dry land. Perhaps dry land is our problem."

With *Waterlog*, Deakins arguably invented the swimoir genre, but it's the depth and breadth of his interests that make the book unique. I do have a writerly bone to pick with him, though. No one can write and swim at the same time, yet it feels like that's exactly what he's doing! Time and again while reading *Waterlog*, I was astounded at his recall of the minutest details of his swimming adventures. It reads almost as if he's swimming as the reader reads. I kept wondering, *how the hell does he do it?*

There are other genres in what might be considered the swimming canon. John Cheever's famous short story "The Swimmer" is cited by nearly every swimoir-ist, though I'm almost embarrassed to say I only got around to reading it recently. Cheever frames the journey as an odyssey with classical echoes, a story that has won acclaim as a great work of short fiction. The protagonist, Ned Merrill, decides to swim back to his home through the pools of his suburban neighbors, a journey that starts out as a lark and slowly turns into a descent into hell. "The Swimmer" is less about swimming than suburban life, but I can see why it has such a strong appeal for those of us who are hopelessly ruled by a need to be immersed in water.

Some of the most compelling writing about swimming has appeared in magazines and blogs. For more than twenty years, Irish swimmer Donal Buckley has recorded advice, information, and open-water swimming news in his widely read LoneSwimmer blog. (It was where I finally learned about cold-immersion diuresis—why one feels the urge to pee right after swimming.) He also gives much space to personal musings, his search through water for "fleeting revelations to inchoate questions I do not know how to articulate," which sounds like more effort to dance about architecture. But for me, the swimmer-writer from whom I've drawn the most inspiration is someone who never wrote a swimoir or a blog: Oliver Sacks, the late neurologist whose towering reputation comes from his work in an entirely different realm.

In his books *Awakenings* and *The Man Who Mistook His Wife for a Hat*, Sacks invented (he would say revived) the genre of literary case studies. Like so many others, I was already a longtime admirer of his work; but for me, encountering his piece "Water Babies" in a 1997 issue of *The New Yorker* was an "Aha!" moment. It changed the way I looked at my own swimming and helped point me toward a way to write about it. "I have never found swimming monotonous or boring," he writes. "There is an essential rightness about swimming, as about all such flowing and, so to speak, *musical* activities.... One can move in water, play with it, in a way that has no analogue with air."

For Sacks, swimming is not mere "exercise," it's a kind of meditative practice. "The mind can float free, become spellbound, in a state like a trance." Swimming, like walking, is a form of daydreaming that's conducive to problem-solving and creativity. The mind can wander without any particular focus, which makes fresh, unexpected connections possible. And it's what's behind the trope that we get some of our best ideas in the shower. I do a lot of my best thinking while I'm in the water, but I have to summon up various mnemonic devices for recall. Then, when I get out, I have to have something ready to write on, which usually gets damp and droopy. In Sacks, I found a kindred spirit: "Sentences and paragraphs would write themselves in my mind, and at such times I would have to come to shore every so often to discharge them...every half hour or so, drippingly, on to paper." (I figure that's also how Roger Deakins must have written most of *Waterlog*.)

Swimming and writing have come to be intimately connected for me, as they were for Sacks. And that's the genesis of this book, a series of snapshots of my own cold-water adventures. It explores some of the myths and facts about the effects of cold water on the body—from my personal experience, but also grounded in science. If you're looking for a how-to book packed with information on the latest research, you'll find some of that here. I don't profess to be an expert in anything but my own experience.

The book gives a glimpse of the burgeoning worldwide

community of open-water and cold-water swimmers, and an account of my own 365-day swim, which garnered more attention than I expected and laid the groundwork for this book. But this is not an inspirational swimoir. It's not about breaking records, overcoming my limitations, or conquering my fears. It's mostly about how I've come to discover—and organize my life around—my desire to fully immerse myself in water on a regular, preferably daily, basis. As far as swimming itself is concerned, I'm really just an everywoman.

One of the pioneers of cold-water swimming, Lynne Cox (about whom you'll read later), sums it up: "On land, I'm a klutz. In the water, I don't have to worry about falling."

CHAPTER 2

Dead Last:
My (not-so-brilliant) swimming career

CHAMPIONS, THEY SAY, start in childhood. And then there's everybody else, the regular kids who play sports mainly for fun and friendship. Nowadays, in the early twenty-first century, we have more enlightened attitudes about sports. Everybody is encouraged to participate, to the best of their ability. Everybody gets to play. When I grew up there was a further subcategory: the klutzes, the wimps, the not-even-remotely-destined-to-be-champions. That's where I fit in.

I had no athletic ability whatsoever. It didn't help that I had so many brothers. They weren't star athletes, but they definitely were jocks, playing on high school football and swim teams. Many sisters develop into high-achieving athletes because they're strongly motivated to keep up with their brothers. I didn't even try. I was clumsy, I was awkward, and I was profoundly risk-averse—due to a freak accident I had as a toddler, in which I lost my left eye.

I was never that interested in team sports, anyway. Somehow, I came to be on my high school basketball team, but never once got called on to play. I have an old photo of myself in my twenties, when I was on a Toronto Island women's softball team called—I'm mortified to say—the Carefree Chiefs. I'm at the plate, swinging the bat, and I look great! It captures one of those moments when I look as though I actually know what I'm doing. What's missing from the photo is how I'd react when a ball was coming at me in the outfield. I'd close my eyes, duck, and cover my head with my arms, anything to avoid reaching up to catch the ball. I do love ice skating. I live in Canada, after all. But though I've been here most of my adult life, I've never played hockey. I can't tolerate the thought of all those bodies whizzing around me, as they gang up on a small, fast-moving, sliding object. When in motion, I need to be on my own.

The one thing that saved me, growing up, was a Great Lake.

As a kid, I had no idea that my neighborhood was an almost ideal place for a would-be swimmer to grow up. When you walk east on almost any street on the grid that is Chicago, you eventually come to the shore of Lake Michigan. In Rogers Park, chances are good there'll be a sand beach to welcome you, which isn't necessarily the case in the rest of the city. Chicago is blessed with a long Lake Michigan coastline, which used to consist of many miles of unbroken beach. As cities became more car-centric in the early twentieth century, it was thought that drivers needed a quick route from downtown to the neighborhoods on the north side of the city. An existing urban expressway called the Outer Drive (later Lake Shore Drive) was extended northward in the 1950s, paving over much of the lakefront and cutting off the neighborhoods from their beaches. Luckily for me, the city stopped laying pavement at Edgewater, more than two miles south of my childhood home. Rogers Park, which sits at the northernmost edge of the city, is still home to an abundance of these street-end beaches.

Growing up, we knew there were families that went on summer vacations, but I can't say we gave it much thought. Those were people with money to spend. We were nine kids, with two parents, and the SUV had yet to be invented—not that we could have afforded one. But the fact that we had a beach at the end of our street was a fact of life. Didn't everybody live a five-minute walk from one of the largest freshwater lakes in the world? Didn't everybody just grab a towel and head down to the water every day in the summer? Really, we had no idea that we lived such a life of privilege. We'd walk east a half-block to busy Sheridan Road, wait for the green stoplight, then walk a couple of blocks to the foot of Touhy Avenue where there was a long expanse of sandy beach stretching to the south. At various points there were short wooden piers extending a few feet into the water to mark the beaches named, by local custom, after the street that ended there: Touhy Beach, Greenleaf Beach, and Farwell Beach, which are now known as Leone Beach, Hartigan Beach, and Loyola Beach.

When I got to be a teenager, I opted for relative solitude on a thin stretch of sand at the end of my street, Chase Avenue. It was on the other side of the breakwater from Touhy, where the crowds and the hot dog stand were, and you had to descend to it on a metal ladder. I think at one time it had been a private beach for the residents of the adjacent apartment building, but over time it shrank and became scruffy and full of pebbles. It was where I went to read and sunbathe by myself, but it's not there anymore. Like many of the street-end beaches, the tiny, anonymous one at the end of Chase Avenue eroded away, surrendering to high water levels and fierce waves.

We often don't retain vivid memories of things that happen on a near-daily basis. That's especially true of summer, when the days seem to dissolve in a haze of sun and heat. So while I know I was there, I don't have many specific memories of being *in* Lake Michigan. Strangely, one of my most vivid memories is an event for which I wasn't even present. I was about seven years old. One day I overheard my brothers talking about an incident at Touhy Beach. Each of my brothers had taken part in the junior lifeguard program run by a man named Sam Leone, an imposing figure who dominated everything that happened at Touhy Beach. My brother Mike was there that day, and he breathlessly described the incident, using a strange word I'd never heard before.

In Mike's telling, it was an extremely hot, sunny day and dozens of people were already on the beach. As Leone was organizing the lifeguards for the morning shift, he noticed something peculiar. The shoreline had moved back, making the beach much bigger. Leone began shouting at the guards to clear everyone off the beach. Mike said he had no idea what was going on, that they were all afraid of Leone's legendary temper. Then Mike and the other junior lifeguards looked out on the water, and saw it: an enormous wave, looming over the beach and moving toward them at high speed. In seconds, water surged over the neighboring athletic field and according to one news account, "sucked two 500-pound [almost 227 kilogram] lifeguard towers into the water like matchsticks."

The strange word was *seiche*: a Great Lakes version of a tsunami that's caused by a sudden shift in air pressure. A violent thunderstorm had passed over the city earlier that morning, and Leone noticed the water marks on the piers showed the lake level had fallen dramatically—6 feet (1.8 meters) or more. Recognizing what was about to happen, Leone shouted at the dumbfounded beachgoers, ordering them to run up the cement ramp to the field house and clearing the beach just in time. Sam Leone was the indisputable hero of the great seiche of 1954. The next day, his picture was on the front page of both Chicago dailies, and when he retired a decade later, Touhy Beach was renamed after him. People at the neighboring beaches to the south weren't so lucky. Some were swept up in the whirlpool and fought their way back to shore. Eight people drowned that day.

The scene my brother described was terrifying, almost unimaginable. I'd seen big waves before, I'd enjoyed diving into and rolling around in them. But a killer wave? How could such a thing happen at the beach I went to almost every day? The thought of that wall of water—more than 10 feet (three meters) high, the news accounts said—rearing up and sweeping people away imprinted on my young mind the tremendous power of water, a knowledge that's lasted all my life. I heard about the seiche second-hand, but the memory of that angry lake has been burned into my brain as vividly as if I'd been there.

I have no memory of learning to swim, but my first clear memory of swimming has defined my life. Early on, I took swimming lessons at the field house near Touhy Beach, and the instructor got it in his head to enroll the whole class in a 100-yard (91.5-meter) race sponsored by the *Chicago Tribune*. The Tribune Meet was a city-wide event that anyone could enter, children as well as adults. Now, you might assume that the notion of every-child-gets-a-gold-star "participant awards" is a contemporary, twenty-first-century phenomenon, but the idea seems to have taken hold, at least in some quarters, as far back as the 1950s. For the Tribune Meet, all you had to do was complete two lengths of the 50-yard (45.7-meter) pool, and you'd get a bronze lapel pin engraved with "Tribune Meet" and the date. The instructor must have figured that all of us were able to meet these modest requirements, but I honestly doubt he was paying close attention to each of us. Like most nine year olds, I had nothing to wear that had lapels, but I really wanted that pin.

My most striking memory of that day is of the sheer size of the outdoor pool. I'd never seen anything like it. It was enormous. Gargantuan. *Huge.* The mother of all pools. As is typical of childhood memories, this one is greatly exaggerated. In fact, I recently managed to find a photo of that very pool on Google. It's still there, adjacent to a municipal field house on California Avenue, and really, it's no big deal—just another large pool. Fifty yards is longer than 50 meters, which I've swum many times, but back then the sight of it was as intimidating as hell, not to mention the hundreds of people sitting in the stands, chattering away as they watched the meet.

How I overcame my initial terror, I have no idea. But I must have, because I did end up in the water. We were divided into successive heats, and I made it to the far end of the pool long after everyone else. I was growing tired as I started the return lap, a now-solitary figure in the enormous pool. It was probably a combination of my laborious pounding of the water and my fierce determination to finish that roused the crowd to start cheering me on. I kept thrashing and pounding the surface of the water and finally made it to the other end. The entire place erupted in applause. I thought it was because people love to root for the underdog. In retrospect, I think they were grateful that the next heat could finally begin.

Yes, I was Dead Last in my heat, possibly in the whole competition. I don't remember much else, not even receiving my bronze lapel pin; but, in time, I also learned there's no humiliation in it. Dead Last was a category I would get used to in my swimming "career." The important thing was to go the distance.

Swimming didn't become such a total preoccupation until I was well into adulthood. My higher education went along a somewhat checkered path but, as I look back, I see that I have never lived far from water. My first year of university was spent at a Catholic college in Milwaukee, Wisconsin, also on Lake Michigan, about 90 miles (almost 145 kilometers) north of Chicago. After that, I transferred to the University of Wisconsin at Madison, the City of Four Lakes—or five, depending on which tourist blurb you read. When I moved to Toronto at the age of 21, I found myself living on another Great Lake, Lake Ontario. When my partner Alec's and my first daughter was six months old, we had a chance to buy a place on Toronto Island. It cost a pittance at a time when the community was threatened with extinction. Now it's the most valuable real estate that nobody can buy. There are many things I could tell you about living in this most unusual of villages, but for the purposes of this book, the main thing is, it gave me ready access to water—just like my childhood in Rogers Park. It mystified me that so many Torontonians were water-shy, even my island neighbors. In spring, I was the first one in the water, and the last one out in the fall. On Toronto Island, my life came into full aquatic bloom.

GOING THE DISTANCE

It may look like I'm trying to create the impression that I'm not a competitive person, but that would be disingenuous. We're all competitive in some way—it's part of human nature—but it only makes sense to pick battles that line up reasonably well with your true abilities. I'm fiercely competitive in more intellectual pursuits—trivia matches, for example. A part of me will always believe that I could have been a champion on *Jeopardy!* (if only you didn't have to push that button so fast!). As far as swimming is concerned, I've always known that my pattern of finishing Dead Last likely would persist throughout my life. I just didn't have the drive to work at swimming, to train, to improve, to "go beyond" and transcend my limits. And yet, the more I became part of the great world-wide group of water lovers, the more I began to think about making a mark of my own. Speed was off the table, but what about endurance? What about slow but steady wins the race? The idea of taking up long-distance swimming in a serious way began to crystallize in my brain. Not crossing the English Channel, mind you, or the 52 miles (83.6 kilometers) of Lake Ontario (which actually has been completed by nearly seventy people since Marilyn Bell first did it in 1954), but I did feel the need for something that would give me a modicum of credibility in the swimming world.

In 2011, an intriguing opportunity presented itself. I was invited to do a reading from one of my plays at a conference in New York City, and it came to my attention that the timing coincided with an event called the Great Hudson River Swim. As I read up on the sponsor organization, NYC Swim, I learned there was a whole universe of swimming competitions open to anyone, not just Olympic-level athletes. To qualify for the Great Hudson River Swim, you just had to pay fifty bucks and show that you were capable of swimming 1,500 meters (almost a mile). Piece of cake! I was ready to (bad pun) dive right in. Signing up would give me a chance to get into open water right in downtown Manhattan. Armed with a qualifying form signed by the lifeguard at my local pool, I booked a plane ticket and headed to the Big Apple.

Race day was lovely—sunny, calm, mild late-May air temperature. I heard some expressions of dismay when the organizers announced that the water temp was 61 F (16 C), but I knew it wouldn't be a problem for me. The actual distance was 2.5 kilometers (about 1.5 miles), slightly longer than I'd done before, but I was pretty sure I'd be fine. All I really wanted to do was finish on my own steam. I was determined to avoid the humiliation of getting hauled into one of the escort boats.

I was one of several hundred swimmers who jumped off Pier 45 in Hudson River Park near Greenwich Village, and swam the distance south to Battery Park, near Tribeca. To my great relief, I arrived at the finish a bit earlier than I expected, but the icing on the cake was this: I finished second in the female age 60–69 class, which, I later found out, was made up of exactly two entrants: myself, and the woman who came in first. Still, it was my first race since I was nine years old, and I won a clear-plastic paperweight with my name on it!

A couple of years later, another opportunity came along, and it was on my home turf. The Toronto Island Lake Swim was held in Lake Ontario, on a 3.8-kilometer (2.4-mile) course lined with big orange buoys. I'd already been doing longer and longer swims and I was confident I could go the distance. I felt pretty great as I swam under the huge inflatable finish-line arch. Yes, it was pretty much a replay of my Dead Last pattern, since there were people who didn't finish the course at all. But in keeping with the practice that prevails in schools these days, I got a participant ribbon.

I started to think about working up to longer and longer swims—5, 7, or 8 kilometers (about 3, 4, or 5 miles). I even conceived of a swim around Toronto Island, a distance of about 10 kilometers (6.2 miles). I would have needed clearance to go through a restricted zone near the island's Billy Bishop Airport, and that quickly put the kibosh on the whole venture. Maybe I could work my way up to trying a section of the legendary 8 Bridges Hudson River Swim, a week-long marathon averaging 18 miles (29 kilometers) per day.

You maybe won't be surprised to learn that none of that came to pass. Now, ten years later, 4 kilometers (about 2.5 miles) is the longest distance I've ever swum. I came to realize that to achieve greater distances, I'd have to capital-T Train. It's the topic serious swimmers talk about all the time: Training. The very word makes me tired. The discipline needed for it is just not in my DNA. In truth, my career as a distance swimmer ended quite ignominiously, as you'll see in a later chapter of this book.

It turned out I had endurance, just not for distance.

My destiny lay in cold. Biting, numbing, chilling cold.

CHAPTER 3

Going Cold:
The making of a psychrolute

It's March. The ice on Lake Ontario is all but gone, confined to a glaze on the rocky shelf at the far end of Ward's Island Beach. As I look at the brilliant blue-green water, my thoughts are irresistibly drawn to plunging in for a nice swim.

Yes, you read that right. Swimming, in Lake Ontario. In March.

Before I go any further, let me make one thing clear: I am not one of those "polar bear" dippers you see on the New Year's Day news, running (screaming and nearly naked) in and out of the water before they've barely had a chance to get wet. No, I am what's known as a "psychrolute," literally one who bathes in cold water. This is not, needless to say, a very large subset of the human population. In fact, pretty much the only place you'll encounter the term is on obscure-word-of-the-day websites, where you'll learn about the Psychrolutes' Society formed by some 19th-century British eccentrics who swam outdoors all winter.

If they were still around today, I'm pretty sure I'd qualify for membership. For a number of years I've been swimming daily in Lake Ontario for the better part of six months of the year, and with global warming I've been extending my season even more. I now swim well into November and on the odd mid-winter day when the sun is strong and the air on the beach is calm.

I know the question you're dying to ask, I've been asked it countless times: Why? As in, why would any sane person deliberately choose to immerse herself in freezing cold water? I can only reply—and I know it's hard to believe—that I do it because I love it. Oh sure, it's a bit daunting when I first wade in. But once I get over the shock of that initial plunge, my body adjusts and I can usually stay in for at least four minutes, depending on the water temperature.

I seem to be one of those people with an unusual tolerance for cold water. Almost as important are the mental factors involved. I often say the word "warm" over and over in my head as I swim, and it seems to do the trick. I never feel cold after swimming, and I've never exhibited any signs of hypothermia. In fact, the main thing I feel when I come out of the water is exhilaration, a sense of being intensely alive.

So, if you're out on the island and you spy a human figure swimming amid the swans and mallards and the odd chunk of ice, don't be alarmed. It's just me, your friendly neighborhood psychrolute.

THIS WAS THE FIRST piece I ever wrote about swimming. It was published in the *Globe and Mail* on March 22, 2006 and was an attempt to coin what I thought was a witty new word: psychrolute. It comes from the Latin *psychrolūtēs*, derived from the ancient Greek ψυχρολουτεῖν, meaning to bathe in cold water. I admit it looks and sounds perilously close to words like "psychopath," "psychosis," and "psychiatric." But thanks to that "r," the word has nothing to do with mental health or people in need of intervention; though it's worth noting that its opposite is psychrophobia, meaning extreme sensitivity and even dread of cold water, a characteristic shared by most normal, sensible humans.

The word appears to have entered the English language in the early nineteenth century when a group of Englishmen formed an organization, the Society of Psychrolutes, to promote the practice of year-round, outdoor swimming. Many of the details about the Society of Psychrolutes have been lost in the mists of time, perhaps due to the fact that it was difficult to record meeting minutes with frozen hands.

The one surviving piece of knowledge specifies that the qualification for membership was a commitment to "the daily practice of bathing out of doors from November to March." An early president of the Society of Psychrolutes was one Sir Lancelot Shadwell, a prominent barrister who "was in the habit of bathing every day, whatever the weather, in one of the creeks of the Thames." It was said that he conducted court proceedings from the water, and on one occasion granted an injunction. (Presumably, he managed not to drip on the paper.)

There is another, more contemporary meaning of the word, which also has to do with the life aquatic. *Psychrolutes marcidus* is the scientific name for a fish that inhabits the deep ocean off the coasts of Australia and New Zealand. But the creature has another name, by which it is much better known: the blobfish. These unfortunate creatures have no muscles, and thus no power to propel themselves through the water. All they can do is float around, aimlessly. Add to that the fact that their gelatin-like mass gives them a lower density at great depths, so they have to stay in the deepest, coldest waters.

Much abuse has been heaped on this unfortunate creature. The ultimate insult came in 2013, when Psychrolutes marcidus was named the world's ugliest animal by the Animal Planet cable channel. To add insult to injury, the blobfish is an endangered species. As of 2015, there were only four hundred and twenty left in the wild. (No idea how they counted.) Nevertheless, the blobfish does have its staunch defenders. There's even a website called Blobfish

Café that promotes respect for this beleaguered creature. One marine scientist claimed that the website appeared to be "nothing more than a prank." The webmaster's name is Donald Shrimpton. You be the judge.

When I first encountered the term psychrolute, I felt an instant kinship, since I check all the same boxes: I swim in cold water, I'm not the sleekest fish in the sea, and there are times when I feel like nothing so much as a gelatinous mass moving through liquid. I've come to accept that my attempts to get the word into mainstream usage will never get off the ground. But I do get asked this question on a near-daily basis: What could possess a person to go into freezing cold water *voluntarily*?

Or, put more simply: Are you *crazy*?

I've always had a high tolerance for the cold, which I suspect is partly genetic. In the dead of winter my father used to go out hatless, the front of his coat unbuttoned. People would say "Mac, how can you stand it?" Now they say much the same to me.

In the early days of my off-season tiptoeing (literally) into Lake Ontario, I drew inspiration from an island neighbor named Klaus Rothfels. He was an esteemed cytogeneticist at the University of Toronto, world-renowned for his work on black flies. Klaus passed away in the late eighties and a scholarship in his name is awarded annually to a graduate student in cell biology at the University of

Toronto. Back then, I didn't really know about his accomplishments. To me, he was Klaus, a vigorous, barrel-chested man with wind-blown, white hair, whom I frequently encountered on Ward's Beach. He used to swim regularly to an arm of land known as the Leslie Street Spit, a round trip of about a mile and a half (almost 2.5 kilometers) through a busy shipping channel. The harbor officials tried to stop him, but eventually gave up. I once asked him if he wasn't afraid of getting hit by a one of the big tankers.

"Oh, no," he replied with a laugh. "I make sure they see me. I just splash around a bit."

Over time Klaus noticed that I was becoming a comrade, going in the lake on a daily basis, even when others found it too cold. He once commented on our shared tolerance for cold water. "You and I are special," he laughed, patting himself on the belly. "We have padding." At the time I thought he was mocking my weight, but I came to appreciate that he was simply stating a fact that's served me well ever since: Skinny people just don't do well in cold water.

My love affair with cold water swimming didn't really get going until I was nearly fifty, when my female body entered the inexorable process known as menopause. For me, "the change" came with the standard panoply of negative effects: mood swings, insomnia, depression, the works. As for hot flashes, what I had weren't intermittent surges of body heat. No, I felt hot *all the time*. Inside, outside, no matter the weather. Raging, unremitting heat, except when I was in the water. Even in normal summer water temperatures of

20 C (68 F) or higher, swimming helped cool me down, though warm weather itself was also a kind of curse. I struggled with depressed moods for years before I learned that "reverse SAD" or summer Seasonal Affective Disorder was a real diagnosis. That, combined with my menopausal turmoil, was what drove me to explore cold-water "treatment" before I even knew there was such a thing.

Autumn, when the lake temperatures started to drop, was my season of relief. Over time, as early winter arrived, I just kept on going, long after everyone else had left the beach. Most days it was just me and the occasional dog. As the water grew colder, I found myself experiencing real freedom—not just from my internal inferno, but from my gloomy outlook and crippling mood swings. Cold water brought back my interest in life. It gave me back my joy.

IT'S ALL ABOUT THE HANDS

One of the deadliest disasters in modern history happened on December 26th, 2004: the tsunami that struck the west coast of Indonesia, killing more than two hundred thousand people. I was still fairly new to full-on cold-water swimming, and got it into my head to do a New Year's Day swim to raise money for the survivors. I announced my plan to my island neighbors, making clear this wasn't going to be the typical run-in-screaming-run-out polar-bear plunge. I asked people to donate their desired amount for every minute I stayed in the water, and said my goal was five minutes. More than fifty people came to Ward's Beach that morning to cheer me on. I invited those assembled to join me in the water, but (surprise, surprise!) there were no takers. They were keen to donate, not to plunge.

With the sun shining and the air calm, I figured staying in for five minutes in my neoprene, shorty suit wouldn't be a problem. And it wasn't. I swam back and forth along the shore, periodically stopping to check in with my friend Joanna on how long I'd been in. When she signaled I'd hit the five-minute mark, I came out of the water. A neighbor carrying a donation bucket shouted that my swim had raised more than $500. I felt exhilarated and, honestly, not particularly cold, except for one part of me. My hands were like bricks, as hard as rocks. Even though I warmed them at the fire someone had built, it was a long time—a half-hour or more—before sensation returned to my fingers.

It was my first experience of what would become a major preoccupation in my cold-water exploits. Among living species, humans have had remarkable evolutionary success (though we seem to be squandering that heritage in our abject failure to fight climate change). The popular assumption is that it's due to our big brains, but anthropologists know the real reason: hands. Our unique, versatile, four-digits-with-opposable-thumb hands. It's a lesson I've had to learn more than once, as you'll see throughout this book. In fact, I've broken a lot of rules and guidelines, in my blissful ignorance. In the early years of this mad habit, I became a kind of cold-water lab rat without really intending to. I'll tell you some of what I've learned, both from experience and plain dumb luck, and I'll pass the baton to some of the actual, qualified experts in the field.

First, a bit of history. Believe it or not, humans voluntarily have been immersing themselves in cold water for an awfully long time.

FROM FOLK WISDOM TO EMPIRICISM

A survey of cold-water immersion practices through the centuries simultaneously yields a kind of capsule history of science itself. Many animals, such as walruses, polar bears, and most fish, thrive in cold water, but we humans understandably are wary of its danger and extreme discomfort. It's hard to think of an activity that screams, "Buyer beware!" more than plunging into freezing cold water; but claims for the health benefits of cold water date back to antiquity. Hippocrates, the great Greek physician, was a proponent of water therapy in general and cold water in particular.

For centuries, claims that cold-water swimming improved human health and well-being were based largely on folk wisdom and anecdotal accounts. That began to change in the late-eighteenth century with the work of Scottish physician James Currie, who used cold water in the successful treatment of a contagious fever in Liverpool. In 1797, he published an influential pamphlet, "Medical Reports on the Effects of Water, Cold and Warm, as a Remedy in Fevers and Other Diseases," that contains the first English record of clinical observations using a thermometer. The practice of sea bathing became popular around the same period, and coastal countries saw the growth of seaside resorts to capitalize on the perceived health benefits of saltwater. In 1846, Victorian physician James Gully published *The Water Cure in Chronic Disease*, describing the pioneering hydrotherapy treatments at his clinic in Malvern, England, where famous patients included Darwin, Charles Dickens, and Florence Nightingale. The hydrotherapy movement crossed the Atlantic in 1866 with the establishment of John Harvey Kellogg's sanitarium in Battle Creek, Michigan.

The popularity of hydrotherapy diminished with the rise of modern medicine, and cold water was consigned to the category of things to be avoided at all costs.

THE COLD-WATER PROFESSOR

I'm glad I didn't see any of Professor Popsicle's TV appearances before I became a cold-water swimmer.

Gordon Giesbrecht, a Canadian physiologist who operates the Laboratory for Exercise and Environmental Medicine at the University of Manitoba, is known internationally for his studies in cold-water immersion. Specifically, he studies the process of thermoregulation in the human body. He's conducted hundreds of cold-water immersion studies that have provided valuable information about cold-stress physiology and pre-hospital care for human hypothermia. Basically, his method is to have his subjects (and, to be fair, himself) sit in tubs of freezing cold water and record various physical reactions during and after they get out. No wonder they call him Professor Popsicle!

More than a scientist, Giesbrecht is very much a public advocate for water safety, which has led him to become a media figure as well. In the early 2000s he began doing video segments for the Discovery Channel on cold-water survival strategies. They were mostly about what to do if you fall through the ice but with added tips, such as how to survive a night in the woods if your snowmobile goes through the ice and sinks. His profile on Discovery led to guest turns on talk shows like *Late Night with David Letterman.* In his home country, Geisbrecht became well-known for his appearances on *The Rick Mercer Report,* a popular weekly series that ran for fifteen seasons on the CBC. Mercer is a Canadian comic known for biting, headline-driven satire. His up-for-anything stunts were a trademark of the series. In their first show together, Mercer had to climb into a tub of ice-cold water for several minutes, while Geisbrecht measured his vitals. On a later episode, he had Mercer drive a car right into a lake to demonstrate the various ways to get out before the vehicle sinks, a segment that simultaneously was hilarious and terrifying. Vehicle submersion is actually one of Geisbrecht's specialties: One of the questions on his website reads, "Where can I buy a center punch for exiting my sinking vehicle?" A center punch? Carpenters know that's a tool that drills a small hole to mark the spot where a drill bit will enter; but in this case, it's used to break a window to enable a quick escape from a sinking car. It retails for less than $20. I guess it's a good idea to have one, if only to remind yourself *not* to drive into a body of water.

There's nothing whimsical about Giesbrecht's website, Cold Water Boot Camp. It's deadly serious, chockablock with terms like "shivering thermogenesis," and charts labeled "When and how you can die in cold water." The site revolves around a technique Giesbrecht has coined the "1-10-1 Rule," which can be summed up as, "If you fall in ice water, you have *one minute* to get control of your breathing, *ten minutes* of meaningful movement, and *one hour* before you become unconscious due to hypothermia." In the first minute it's crucial to keep your head above water and control your breathing to prevent hyperventilating. Focus on taking long, deep breaths. For the next ten minutes you have the ability to take action to make yourself safe before nerves and muscles stop responding. Finally, you have about an hour before hypothermia sets in, possibly a bit more if you are wearing a lifejacket. In essence, Professor Popsicle has filled a generation of Canadians with terror at the thought of going near, not to mention *in*, cold water.

Something else that stokes fear in Canadians is ice rescue videos: staged scenarios featuring guys in yellow survival suits that local TV stations run at the start of winter. They usually end with the same warning: "No ice is safe ice." This doesn't keep people from going out onto the ice for fun and sport. People who do wild skating (on, for instance, the Toronto Island lagoon system, as many of us do) know to carry safety gear, and learn the technique of hoisting oneself out of the water and onto safer ice. Here in Canada and other northern climes, there's snowmobiling and ice fishing on frozen lakes. But with climate change, thaw-and-freeze cycles play havoc with the usual patterns, and result in more frequent emergency rescues. Then there are people who rush out onto the ice to try to rescue their dogs. The sad fact is that the owner is more likely to die than the animal.

The key variable in these cold-water scenarios, though, is that they're about *involuntary* entry: situations in which a person or persons have ended up in freezing water accidentally as the result of a mishap. And the water doesn't have to be freezing to be lethal, as a terrible incident in Ontario's Algonquin Park demonstrated. A canoe overturned in choppy water in Lake Opeongo, leaving three men clinging to the craft. Some kayakers saw the accident and paddled over to help. They were able to pull two of the men to shore and told them to start a fire. By the time they returned to the canoe, the third man was lacking vital signs, and later was pronounced dead at the hospital. It was mid-October, and the water was still well above freezing, about 10–12 C (50–54 F), but the third man had been in the water too long. Prolonged immersion in cold water definitely is not something to be messed with.

I've never fallen into cold water, but I know people who have, and lived to tell the tale. Still, the alarmism of Professor Popsicle and yellow-suited rescue crews don't tell the whole story. There's a world of difference for people who go into cold water by choice, and there are specific situations in which humans have developed remarkable cold-water tolerance. There are, of course, elite swimmers such as Lewis Pugh and Lynne Cox, who I discuss in a later chapter. Another famous example is the mostly-female ama pearl divers of Japan, whose thicker layer of body fat helps them endure cold water during long periods of diving. They are also free divers, with the ability to hold their breath for up to two minutes. The scientific understanding of these unusual humans is growing, along with the discovery that they may not be so unusual after all. While their extraordinary abilities partially can be attributed to the vagaries of genetics, there's new research demonstrating that even ordinary schmucks can achieve cold-water bragging rights, and do it within the boundaries of safety.

CHAPTER 4

Kill and Cure:
The science of cold immersion

BECAUSE HUMANS ARE terrestrial creatures, not aquatic (though the ama pearl divers might be an exception), the bulk of our science on human adaptation to cold has concerned itself with cold *climate* rather than cold water. It's a bit of a mystery that humans have any ability to tolerate cold at all, since the scientific consensus is that Homo sapiens migrated out of the tropical environment of Africa thousands of years ago. Some researchers lean toward the view that our cold adaptabililty stems from genetic material handed down to us by our Neanderthal ancestors. It's fairly well-established that there was cross-breeding in Europe between modern humans and Neanderthals, though there is still fierce resistance from those heavily invested in the notion that nature has a hierarchy, and we're at the top. Personally, though I'm intrigued by the idea that my cold-water fixation comes from a smidgen of Neanderthal DNA,

I lack the expertise to engage in such discussions. I'm no slouch in absorbing the essence of scientific studies—I've had to do it many times in my career—but the subject of the human body in cold water is complex, and the research is rapidly evolving. I need lay translation, and I'm glad a growing body of research is bridging that gap.

In recent years, groundbreaking work in cold-water immersion has been carried out at the University of Portsmouth in the UK. These studies bring a very different perspective from that of Geisbrecht and other experts, whose focus is disaster prevention. Michael Tipton is a professor of human and applied physiology at the University of Portsmouth. His colleague, Heather Massey, studies human physiological responses to cold and other extreme conditions. In addition to being researchers, both Tipton and Massey are athletes: Tipton is an ironman triathlete; Massey is a seasoned cold-water swimmer who completed a solo crossing of the English Channel in 2019. The fact that they are both scientists and active participants in their subject of study gives their work a real-life applicability, acknowledging both the risks of cold-water immersion and the fact that people want to do it anyway. (Combining her passions, Massey sometimes swallows wireless thermometer capsules so she can monitor her body temperature during swims.) In 2017, Tipton, Massey, and several of their Portsmouth colleagues co-authored a comprehensive review of the current research on cold-water immersion, examining the evidence for its benefits in the area of mood disorders, immune function and other health conditions. The journal article's title is "Cold water immersion: kill or cure?" and the answer, of course, is it's both. The authors admit that, at present, the evidentiary basis for *kill* is somewhat more developed than that for *cure*, but their conclusion—far from a simple-minded "stay out of the water"—is that more study is needed on the benefits, as well as the hazards.

In early 2021, Massey and Tipton took part in a webinar on cold-water safety where they presented their research and answered questions in language accessible to non-scientists. They demystified topics that preoccupy many discussions on swimming websites, such as this quote: "White fat is utilised by the body first by conversion to glycogen, thence into glucose for fueling the muscles. However, brown fat is rapidly metabolised to generate heat." Kind of makes your eyes glaze over, doesn't it? Mine certainly do, so I was glad to hear Tipton basically dismiss the whole "brown fat" discussion as not very important. Still, their presentations left the audience of swimmers plenty to be wary of. Massey discussed an alarming condition called swimming-induced pulmonary edema (SIPE) that can arise from any number of cold-water situations, including overly tight wetsuits. Tipton set out to debunk some of what he called the "flawed beliefs" circulating among cold-water devotees, in particular the idea that swimmers can extend their habituation to the cold for longer and longer periods. In fact, Tipton says, repeated exposure to cold water can produce what he termed a "hypothermic" adaptation, in which the acclimated individuals shiver little or not at all, and paradoxically feel comfortable even as their deep body temperature falls. In other words, some open-water swimmers—particularly those who are well acclimatized to cold—can lose the ability to judge how cold their bodies actually are.

Tipton gives the chilling example (no pun intended) of Jason Zirganos, a legendary marathon swimmer who completed four progressively faster crossings of the English Channel in the early 1950s. He was the first person to complete the Triple Crown of Open Water Swimming, which, besides the English Channel, includes crossing the Catalina Channel in California and circumnavigation of Manhattan Island. There's some controversy over his Manhattan Island swim, with reports that toward the end he had to be pulled from the water almost completely unconscious. Like so many elite swimmers, he was always determined to outdo himself, and in 1959 he embarked on a 35-kilometer (almost 22-mile) swim across the North Channel from Ireland to Scotland, in water around 13 C (55 F).

At no time during the swim did he claim to feel cold, yet Zirganos had to be pulled from the water again. He was in the throes of hypothermia and despite efforts to revive him, he later died. In Tipton's words, Zirganos "swam to unconsciousness" because, over time, his body had lost the physical signal that he was getting too cold.

Over the years, I've noticed some version of this in myself. You can get almost *too* used to cold water. From the first time your body tries to tell you—very sensibly—that it doesn't *want* to be there, and through regular immersion, you unlearn that series of reactions. Zirganos' fateful outcome wouldn't happen nowadays with all the safeguards, medical backup, and monitoring that accompanies high-level competitive swims. But with the burgeoning popularity of cold-water practices, Tipton's watchword is more pertinent than ever: "Don't trust how you feel, if you feel okay." Even elite swimmers like Jaimie Monahan, who's done several of the coldest swims every recorded, echoed this advice to newcomers on a recent webinar: "Go by time in the water, not distance."

Of course, people who live in cold latitudes who've been going in cold water for centuries, will continue as they always have, without financial motives or the blessing of science: crazy Swedes jumping in and out of freezing water from their saunas; Russians dousing themselves with buckets of cold water; hardy Brits who frequent Hampstead Heath Ponds year-round. I'm a member of this world-wide clan, and for a long time, I didn't even know it.

NEWS YOU CAN USE

When I started out, I had no idea that what I was doing was a "thing." Social media soon brought me up to speed, where I found a number of like-minded swimming groups. The most prominent was, and still is, the Outdoor Swimming Society (OSS), founded in the early 2000s by British journalist Kate Rew to encourage people to rediscover the joys of swimming in rivers, lakes, and other wild bodies of water. The OSS, which has grown to an online reach of over half a million, has spearheaded a wave of change in the way outdoor swimming is viewed, and the number of people who take part in it. They have a subgroup for what they call winter swimmers, who have their own motto: *E Frigore Robur!* "From cold comes strength."

Keep in mind that this book is a sharing of my experiences, in which I've served as my own guinea pig, finding my way largely through trial and error—some of which you'll read about later on. As I emphasized earlier, don't expect to find a handbook or how-to of cold-water swimming in these pages; but for readers thinking of dipping a toe or more in cold water, I've done a bit of legwork for you, cobbling together information and advice from experts and trustworthy sites. So, here begins the "news you can use" section of this book.

I can't think of a better place to start than with a quote from the "Getting Started" section of the OSS website:

> Simply start swimming in summer when the water is nice and warm. Come Autumn, just keep going. Among swimmers, this is known as "riding the thermometer down." The golden rule: don't overdo it—there's always tomorrow. When you feel cold, get out, get dressed and warm up. You'll find your tolerance, both time and temperature, will steadily improve. Safety is paramount. While it's important to observe all precautions normally associated with swimming in open water, low temperatures mean taking

extra care. Don't start cold training until spring/ early summer when the water temperature is at least 15C. Never jump or dive into water below 15C (59F). Always wade or lower yourself in— this gives your body time to switch into "cold mode." Avoid having cold water enter your nose. There is very little bone between the nasal cavity and your brain, and chilling the brain can result in cold shock. Always wear a swim cap, as a surprisingly large amount of body heat is lost through the head. A brightly coloured cap will also enhance your visibility, which you can increase further with the use of a brightly coloured tow float.

I say a hearty amen to everything here, especially about wearing a cap. There's a spot on the very top of my head that throbs like crazy when the water temp is below about 10 C (50 F). My face hurts in cold water, too, but little can be done about that. You can keep your head up if you swim breaststroke, a stroke I've always found very awkward. The OSS says goggles are optional, but for me they're mandatory. I'm monocular and I need to take extra care of the one working eye I have. And for newbies to open water, a tow float is a kind of thick-walled balloon on a long cord attached to your waist. I put off getting one because I thought it would be a literal drag, but honestly, I hardly feel it when I'm swimming. And it really does increase visibility when there are fast-moving watercrafts around. Some models serve as dry bags, if you close them up tightly enough, so you can carry small items like eyeglasses, a wallet, or a cell phone (though you'd be wise to put valuables in a second sealable bag inside the tow float).

GETTING IN, GETTING OUT

How's this for contradictory advice? Go *quickly*, but *slowly*. It makes perfect sense when you break it down into steps: Don't delay getting into the water. Don't stand around on shore in your swimsuit, chatting. Don't think too much. Don't give yourself time to get cold beforehand. Just *get in* but do it slowly to avoid what's called the "cold-shock response," caused by rapid cooling of the skin. The cold-shock response is a range of reactions in the body, including narrowing of the blood vessels (vasoconstriction) as well as an increase in heart rate and blood pressure. The cold-shock experience begins with gasping and hyperventilating, as blood moves toward the middle of the body in a bid to keep warm. I know it's fun to run and scream like they do at the New Year's polar-bear dips, but seriously, folks: Walk in slowly. And don't dive into cold water head-first. It's much safer, not to mention more enjoyable, to get into the water slowly. By splashing your torso and face before you immerse, you can control your breathing and help prevent more serious reactions.

Stay within your depth. It's not a hard and fast rule, since bodies of water and ways to access them vary so much; but it's good advice because it keeps you close to shore, so you can get out quickly. Getting *out* of the water is, if anything, more important than getting in. You need an exit strategy. Make sure you work out how you're going to get out of the water before you go in. There's an all-too-obvious corollary to that rule: Make sure you *can* get out of the water. It's not as stupid as it sounds as I've learned, the hard way, on more than one occasion. One day, during a period when the water level of Lake Ontario was quite high, I decided to have a swim off a concrete wall that runs along the eastern edge of the island. It used to be a boat landing, but all that's left is a couple of crumbling stone steps. There's no ladder, but with the high water I figured I'd have no trouble scrambling onto the steps; except for the fact that I *did* have trouble. I miscalculated the height of the lowest step and couldn't quite manage to lift myself. I wasn't in danger because the water wasn't terribly cold, and I knew there were people within shouting distance. But I was too embarrassed to yell for help. I managed to hoist myself out, but it took many attempts and longer than it should have. Plus, I must have looked ridiculous, lying on the concrete on my stomach like a beached whale.

THE THREE WS: WATER, WEATHER, WIND

I know this book is about swimming, but surprisingly, the temperature of the water may be the least of your concerns. What's going on above and around you can be just as challenging as the cold water itself. In winter, the freezing air temperature cause ice to build up on shorelines, making entry and exit points treacherous. When the ice on Ward's Beach builds up past a certain point, I have to stop. It's just near-impossible to get close to open water and scramble over mounds of crusty ice. Floating sheets can cut your skin. One year the lake froze like glass all the way to the Leslie Street Spit, about 1.5 kilometers (a mile) from Ward's Island. No swimming, but the glorious skating conditions more than made up for it.

I've said it before (mostly on Facebook groups) and I'll say it again: The real enemy of the winter swimmer is *wind*. I've never let a fierce wind keep me out of the lake, but I really, really hate it when there's a 35-mile-per-hour westerly blowing as I walk out into the water. As one blogger wrote, "There is nothing worse than standing half out of the water, trying to convince yourself to finish getting wet, while the wind whistles across all the exposed damp skin." The weird thing about wind is, once you're in the water you hardly even feel it. Then you have to come out again, and the longer your hands are exposed to the wind, the harder it is to get yourself dressed.

HOW LONG SHOULD YOU STAY IN?

I could be flippant and say, not long enough to freeze solid or you won't be able to get out, but it's a serious question, one that comes up more frequently than any other. The answer is that frustrating phrase: "It depends." The experts don't agree—in fact, they don't even agree on whether they *should* agree. Heather Massey is reluctant to lay down hard and fast rules: "What works for one person is not appropriate for another…. The best thing to do is to be aware of your body's responses to cooling: Are you shivering? Can you coordinate your stroke? Is it as efficient as usual? Do you feel vague or off-kilter? If the answer is yes to any of these questions, it is time you were out of the water."

Tipton is somewhat more prescriptive. In an online seminar he stated that swimmers should stay in cold water for 10–15 minutes, with an outside maximum of 20 minutes. He reinforces this rule by recommending swimmers monitor their time in the water, if necessary with a watch or other waterproof timepiece. People who engage in extreme outdoor activities tend to be stubborn individualists who don't take kindly to rules and hate being told what to do. Massey's follow-your-instincts approach has become more common among swimmer-scientists. Taken together, the two views are a paradox: Follow your instincts, but *don't* follow your instincts. So, yes, it's complicated. A lot of things in human life are paradoxical. In essence, I don't think Tipton and Massey really contradict one another. In different ways, they both attempt to address the inherent tension between *can* and *should*. Many people say they begin cold-water swimming to stretch themselves, go beyond their limits. Tipton's message is a continual reminder that the human body has very real limits in its ability to deal with cold water. They may vary from person to person and they can change with time and circumstances. We ignore them at our peril. Massey says as much when she advises swimmers "not to set time or distance goals which encourage you to stay in longer than you would want."

I've found this to be the case in my personal evolution. From my earliest days of cold-water swimming, I've experienced an odd sensation of internal warmth. It's not just that I'm "getting used to" the temperature—that happens within a few of minutes of entering the water. This warming sensation comes on when I've been in the water for at least 15 minutes, and it's especially noticeable when the water temperature is between 8 and 11 C (46 and 52 F). I feel completely normal, I'm enjoying myself and I almost feel like I can stay in the water indefinitely. When that hits, I know it's time to start getting out. No frantic rush, I just start heading back to shore. At first, I figured it was my brain playing a trick on me, making me think the water wasn't really cold at all. It was always a bit mysterious, but I had enough sense to listen to it. You might say I trusted my instinct to *not* trust my instinct about how long to stay in. I think now that it's a version of what Tipton described with the Greek swimmer Jason Zirganos, and I realize that without knowing it, I was following his rule: "Don't trust how you feel, if you feel okay." It's one of the ways I've been lucky in my personal trial-and-error ways.

In layperson's language, Tipton's conclusion might be summed up thusly: The more acclimatized you are to the cold, the less able your brain is to properly assess how long you should stay in the water. As I get older, I find myself coming around even more to his advice about timing. In water below about 10 C (50 F), I decide beforehand how long I'm going to stay in, and stick to it. It's a loose correlation of water temp and minutes: 5 C (41 F) means no more than five minutes in the water. I don't wear a watch, so I literally count the minutes. It takes my mind off the cold.

As the water temp creeps down to near-freezing, I tend to do less swimming and more head-above-water dipping.

During the course of the Covid-19 winter, I've adopted a new timekeeping practice: singing! I'm serious. I have a repertoire of folk ballads, mostly Irish (I sometimes sing them on dry land, too). I know just how long they last, so I can repeat or cut verses as needed, and I've found it to be a happier way than counting to distract myself from the cold. Mind you, most of these old ballads are not what you would call happy-go-lucky songs. Many have to do with unrequited love, death, and other grim topics. There's even an element of danger in some of them, like the Irish tune "The Hare's Lament," which recounts a hunt from the doomed rabbit's point of view. I think that singing it might be relaxing, while simultaneouly keeping me on my guard in the cold water. There's another tune called "My Boy Willie," a women's lament for her lover, who drowns at sea. That one seems particularly pertinent.

HYPOTHERMIA: IT'S NOT HYPE

What is hypothermia? You don't really want to know, at least not from first-hand experience. I did experience it once, and not in the circumstances you might expect. More about that later. Most people think it's like feeling really cold, shivering, etc. Not even close. Hypothermia creeps up. It begins when the body's core temperature drops below 37 C (98.6 F), and persistent shivering is only the first sign, followed by reduced dexterity in hands, and difficulty using the lips and tongue to speak. Those who swim regularly in open water often experience mild pre-hypothermia symptoms, such as feeling their hands stiffen. Particularly in winter, even mild symptoms can be dangerous. If you can't use your hands to get dressed, or are shivering too hard to put your clothes on or drink your tea, you risk getting even colder and increasing the hypothermia symptoms. The best way to avoid the worst symptoms is to get out of the water before you start to feel cold. You can learn to feel at what point this happens for you. By wearing a watch, you can note your safe exposure time. Even the shortest open-water dip in winter will cause your body temperature to fall, and it is very difficult to warm up after swimming when the air is just as cold, if not colder, than the water.

As soon as you get out of the water, you should direct your energies immediately toward getting dressed. To help restore your warmth, bring a woolly hat, socks, and gloves, plus lots of small, loose layers without fiddly zips and hooks. Go for slippery, slidey clothes—nothing tight: easy on, easy off. Jeans, leggings, and materials like Lycra are not your friends after winter dips. Avoid anything with buttons because you can't button fast enough. Zippers require too much dexterity. Go for snaps—they're the easiest to maneuver with frozen hands. (There I go, harping on hands again.) Dry robes, also known as changing robes, are ubiquitous in cold-water swimming circles. They are large and tent-like, with enough room underneath to change from a wet swimsuit into dry clothes. I've never felt the need to invest in one, since my old, extra-puffy, down parka does the job just fine.

Once you're dressed, get moving!

AFTERDROP

Cold-water swimmers have a mysterious lingo, and this is a word you'll hear more than any other. (I experienced it before I knew it had a name.) What swimmers call after-drop is exactly that: a drop in body temperature that occurs *after* you get out of the water. At first you feel fine, then you start to get colder, sometimes growing faint, shivering violently and feeling unwell. This happens because when you swim, your body shuts down circulation to your skin, pooling warm blood in your core. This process helps you stay in the water longer. With reduced circulation to your peripheries, skin, and subcutaneous fat is turned into a thermal layer, akin to a natural wetsuit. Marathon swimmers have a pet name, bioprene, for this fat layer. But as you start to warm up, the process reverses: blood starts to recirculate in your extremities and peripheral blood vessels, cooling as it travels. Tipton's research shows a swimmer's core body temperature can drop by as much as 4.5 C (8 F), bringing on shivering or hypothermia, and feeling faint and unwell.

Warmup is a subject of much discussion on cold-water swimming sites. The general consensus is to warm up slowly, perhaps with a warm drink, but not to rush the process by having a hot shower or bath, which can cause low blood pressure and fainting. People share their practices and tips, many of which involve getting into their cars and turning on the heat. Lately I've seen a new twist: Leave a thermal blanket in the car—or even an electric blanket, plugged in. It's only recently that I've come to appreciate how unusual my own situation is. One of the main suggestions for rewarming is exercise, and I've got that one down pat. I have no choice but to walk, briskly, back to my house, which takes seven to nine minutes, then run a nice hot bath. It was a habit that formed from the beginning, though I know now it goes against the gradual rewarming recommendation of the OSS and other cold-water groups—yet another rule I broke in my ignorance. Still, I've never suffered any ill consequences, probably because the rewarming process is already well underway during my walk home from the beach. As for afterdrop, I've only experienced it a few times, and hardly ever shiver anymore.

TO WETSUIT OR NOT TO WETSUIT?

It's a completely personal choice. Whatever you decide, don't feel guilty about it. As Heather Massey says, "It isn't cheating to wear neoprene." In the early days of my cold-water obsession, I wore a "shorty" wetsuit, which was sleeveless and knee-length. Contemplating my 356-day swim in 2016, I wondered whether I might need to graduate to a full-body wetsuit. Many cold-water swimmers wear them. So I tried one, once, and I absolutely *hated* it. Hated the time it took to put it on, hated yanking it over my skin, hated peeling it off. But most of all, I hated the way it cut me off from direct contact with the water. As Roger Deakins wrote, a wetsuit "cannot approach the sensuality of swimming in your own skin." In fact, that's what swimming without a wetsuit is called: "going skins" or, in the more risqué sectors of the swimming world, "going naked."

Some open-water competitions allow wetsuits, others don't. But the hardcores go by English Channel rules: swimsuit, cap, and goggles, that's it. That's my own preference nowadays. Since I don't have to follow any rules, I do make one concession: neoprene gloves, 5-millimeter (0.2-inch) thickness. Yep, there's that hand fetish again! I want to feel the cold water while making sure I don't lose sensation in my hands.

BREAKING THE CARDINAL RULE

I always dread it when this topic comes up: "Never swim alone." You'll see it on all the open-water sites. It's good advice. It's almost the cardinal rule of open-water swimming. So let me confess right here, right now, that I break it on a near-daily basis. And the not-so-well-kept secret in the open-water community is this: I've got lots of company, prominent company, at that. There's Donal Buckley, the Irish swimmer and blogger. He calls himself the "Prophet of Cold," and publishes the world's most popular open-water swimming blog. The name of his blog? LoneSwimmer. Buckley is very plugged in to the open-water world, supporting all kinds of competitions and group swims. But when it comes to his personal practice—well, let's see: He's swum the English Channel, he lives right by the ocean in County Waterford, and swims regularly at spots he knows very well. As he explains, "The name arose because, contrary to Open Water Rule Number One, *Never Swim Alone*, by necessity most of my swimming was by myself."

It's the same for me: When I started swimming in cold

water, I couldn't find anyone who wanted to join me. On the OSS website a few years back, someone started a discussion thread on the question: "Do you ever swim alone?" It developed into a major confessional for many people, who sheepishly admitted they swam solo. Many gave reasons along the lines of, "If I always had to go with a companion I'd hardly ever swim," and stressed their own cautionary practices: only going solo in bodies of water they know well, and staying close to shore; making sure others know where they are, and how long they'll be gone; keeping abreast of conditions on currents and tides.

Roger Deakins broke the rule for almost the entirety of his legendary swim around Britain, as documented in *Waterlog*. One of the glories of the book is the way he conjures up the experience of being in the water, absorbed in his thoughts and his surroundings, beautifully, swimmingly alone. Deakins took risks on his swimming odyssey—dealing with strong currents and fierce undertows, and sharing a shipping channel used by barges and other large vessels. He even tried swimming down the Hell Gill Force waterfall, but changed his mind and managed to claw his way back to the top. He admits to his own foolishness, later wisely deciding against a solo plunge into Scotland's Gulf of Corryvreckan, one of the world's most fearsome whirlpools. But Deakins never second-guessed his decision: Given the nature of the task he set himself, it's unlikely the question of whether or not to go solo even occurred to him.

Still, if social media is any indicator, the majority of open- and cold-water swimmers prefer to swim in groups, for motives that are as much about sociability as safety. And please don't think I'm some kind of misanthrope. There's a modest cohort of regular swimmers here on Toronto Island. We often end up on the beach at the same time and love to chat after our swims, commenting on the waves and speculating on the water temperature. When I've traveled, it's been crucial to connect with other swimmers who generously showed me the ropes. The worldwide community of open-water aficionados is truly a wonderful thing. A quote from one of the group of canal swimmers in Paris sums it up: "La nage en eau froide est un accélérateur d'amitié." *Swimming in cold water is an accelerator of friendship.*

But overall, swimming in groups is not my thing. I don't like the idea of having to gather at a specific time or travel to a beach when I have one practically at my doorstep. In my neck of the woods, there's a particular jones for sunrise swims. I love seeing the gorgeous photos, and sometimes I wish could be there too. But I'm a writer with full-on night-owl tendencies. At this point in life, I'm not up to changing my ways. In fact, the freedom to get in the water whenever I want is part of what makes swimming so vital to my life and well-being. On the occasions when I take part in group swims, I become self-conscious, watching the other swimmers, comparing my speed with theirs, feeling inadequate because I'm usually—surprise, surprise—bringing up the rear. Most swimmers love the social aspects of open water, but I don't feel the bond. I want to be absorbed in my own thoughts and sensations.

I'm probably sounding a bit like Greta Garbo: "I vant

to be alone." In actual fact, I'm rarely truly alone during my swims. Ward's Beach is well-used by the locals, especially walking with their dogs (that occasionally try to "rescue" me). I used to swim far out from shore and loved the feeling of being alone in a large body of water. But when personal watercrafts such as Jet Skis and Sea-Doos became popular, I realized I couldn't hear them approaching the way I could conventional motorboats, especially not with my head halfway under water. Even though I wore the requisite brightly colored swim cap and, more recently, pulled an equally brightly colored towfloat behind me, I was wary of those aquatic hot-rodders sneaking up on me. Nowadays, I stay close to shore, especially when the water is cold. I always know I can get out of the water any time I want. You may not have believed me when I said earlier that I am risk-averse, but it's true.

There's still so much to be learned about the practice of cold-water swimming, and the more people are getting into it, the more we need to learn. But since early 2020, the phenomenon has been affected by something most of us never saw coming: a worldwide pandemic.

CHAPTER 5

Concrete and Chlorine:
The tyranny of the pool

IT'S NOT THAT I have anything against pools. I've swum in plenty of them. They'll do in a pinch. For competitive swimmers they make perfect sense—separated lanes; straight lines on the bottom; water sanitized to kill bacteria and other undesirable critters—everything is controlled, predictable. And there's the rub. That's precisely what those of us who prefer to swim in open, natural, *wild* water are trying to get away from. But in the modern world, pools have become the default option, and the pool mentality intrudes where it doesn't belong.

Some years ago, I found myself back in Chicago in the height of summer. It had been a long time since I'd been in my hometown during swimming season, and I was excited to immerse myself again in the waters of Lake Michigan. It would be a pilgrimage to the very source of my swimming passion. My private beach was long gone, the point of entry paved over by, yes, a parking lot. But one block south, Touhy Beach (as I still thought of it) was still there. The day was calm, the water warm, and I headed in, anticipating a nice, long swim. A Big Swim. I was into distance swimming at the time and thought I'd make a round-trip between Touhy and Farwell Beach, a good half-dozen city blocks to the south.

There was a lifeguard in a rowboat a little way out from shore. I nodded to him as I waded past the boat, on my way into the deeper water where I could commence my big swim. I dove in and my stroke quickly settled into a nice, steady rhythm. As I neared the first of some short wooden piers, a lifeguard boat appeared in front of me, blocking my progress. I tried to swim around it, but he rowed in front of me again. I stopped swimming and faced him, standing in water that was no more than shoulder-deep.

"Something wrong?"

"You're not allowed to swim lengths here, ma'am."

"Lengths? What do you mean, lengths?"

He just shook his head at my question.

"Sorry, ma'am. Swimming lengths isn't allowed here."

"You mean, I can't keep swimming in this direction?"

"That's right, ma'am. You have to stay in this area."

"Why? It's not very deep here. I'm a good swimmer."

"We have to keep an eye on everyone in the water, ma'am. You're not allowed to swim lengths here."

Again with the lengths! Not only was I not permitted beyond the pier, it appeared I was only allowed to bob up and down in a narrowly defined area. I've been "ma'amed" before by lifeguards at my home beach in Toronto, and I usually try to keep my cool. But it was all I could do to keep from yelling at him. "This isn't a pool, it's a lake, a BIG lake and I'm going to swim in it!"

Was I asking for trouble? Would he call the other lifeguards to pull me out of the water? I acquiesced and swam a few strokes back the way I'd come, then swam a few strokes the opposite way, curious to see if this short back-and-forth distance fit his definition of "lengths." Of course, to show me who was boss, he inched the boat as close as he could, without hitting me with an oar. We went on like this for several minutes, a few strokes, going a bit farther each time, then turning back the other way, the lifeguard maneuvering the boat so that it was never more than two or three feet away.

Finally, I'd had enough. I'd come to the motherlode, the original source of my Great Lakes swimming passion, and all I'd managed to do was get a bit wet—and be treated to a demonstration of how the act of swimming had become distorted, synonomous with lengths of a chlorine-filled, concrete hole in the ground. It's yet another way humans turn away from the natural world, and foolishly insist that the experience of being in water can be replaced or, worse, improved upon.

It wasn't always this way. There was a time when swimming in natural bodies of water was considered completely normal.

MOATS, SWIMMING HOLES, AND POOLS

You might think pools are a modern invention, but they go back several millennia. As far as historians know, the Great Bath at the site of Mohenjo-Daro in modern-day Pakistan was the first human-created pool, dug during the third millennium BC. This brick-lined pool was about 39 by 23 feet (about 12 by 7 meters) and likely used for religious ceremonies. UNESCO has designated it a World Heritage Site. Ancient Greece and Rome also had extensive public baths that were central to community life, as meeting places for socializing and relaxing. Later, the Romans built artificial pools in gymnasiums that were used for nautical and military exercises; and Roman emperors had private pools in which they kept fish, hence one of the Latin words for a pool is *piscina*.

These early pools were used as healing baths for various conditions. Swimming took place in natural bodies of water. The Romans built baths in other parts of the empire too, including the one that gave its name to the city of Bath, England, circa 70 AD. The original Roman Bath was a renowned healing spa and swimming locale until well into the twentieth century, when a deadly pathogen was discovered in the water. The historic structure is now for tourist viewing only, replaced for swimming with more modern facilities. It's one example of what Roger Deakins discovers on his epic swim across Britain, lamenting the abandonment and decay of many traditional bathing sites. *Waterlog* traces the history of swimming in Britain, and its evolution from natural swimming holes to contained, human-made structures. Digging moats for defense rather than recreation became common in Britain from the late Middle Ages. Deakins started his journey from a spring-fed moat on his property in Suffolk. Typically, he would swim from place to place, then walk back to retrieve his clothes and gear at the starting point, basically the opposite of doing lengths. (So there, Touhy lifeguard!)

The early twentieth century cemented (pun intended) the transition to enclosed swimming structures, and dozens of open-air lidos were built across Britain. For the most part these lidos were much bigger than modern pools, such as the massive, art deco Jubilee Lido in Cornwall, and they typically designated separate areas or times for men and women to swim. Mixed bathing only became common from the mid-twentieth century. Traditionally, many lidos were open right through the winter, and situated by the seaside to capture seawater in the enclosure. There's an example of this practice in my hometown of Toronto. Built in 1922, the Sunnyside Bathing Pavilion is almost twice the length of an Olympic-sized pool and has room for two thousand bathers. Its Gus Ryder Pool, a concrete behemoth, is filled with several tons of chlorinated water and sits right next to a Lake Ontario beach—an almost perverse turning away from its own environment. As Roger Deakins said of pools, they are "simulations of nature with the one essential ingredient—wildness—carefully filtered out."

With the worldwide growth in the popularity of pools came the need for better sanitation measures. Originally, they employed archaic filtration systems that required their filters, and the water itself, to be changed frequently. By the time of the polio scare in the late 1930s and 1940s, a panic arose over public fears that children could be exposed to the poliovirus in community swimming pools. In 1946, however, a study showed that chlorine was one of the few known chemicals that could kill the virus. As the problem of polio transmission receded, swimming pools regained their popularity as fun and exciting summer venues for families. Moreover, chlorine, as a polio disinfectant, became the near-universal method of pool sanitation, and by the early sixties strict regulations on chlorine in pools were in place.

ENTER THE PANDEMIC

I remember standing in line with my fifth-grade classmates as we waited to get our polio shots. I knew that throughout history there had been terrible epidemics, like the Black Death, when people dropped dead in the streets (which was actually more the case with cholera than the Plague). Like most people who grew up in the twentieth century, that was pretty much the extent of my acquaintance with serious contagious disease.

So when the Covid-19 pandemic and the worldwide lockdown hit in early 2020, I wasn't terribly phased by it, at least on a personal level. Shelter in place? No problem. My spouse and I already worked from home. In fact, much of this book was written during that time. Social distancing? No problem there, either. On this part of the island our houses are close together, sometimes a bit *too* close together, so we don't feel isolated. Like everyone else, we stayed separate from our daughters and grandchild, but FaceTime and outdoor visits made up for that. Get outside once a day for exercise? Let's see, I live in a village on the edge of a nature park, and we're surrounded by water. I venture outside, walk less than five minutes and I'm in the lake. Even in the time of Covid isolation, there couldn't be a better situation for a swimmer. As time went on, though, I realized just how extraordinary my situation was, how truly fortunate I was.

I saw posts by fellow open-water swimmers going through withdrawal, lamenting that they couldn't get to the water since the parks and beaches in Toronto were closed. It was just the time of the season when cold-water swim groups were gearing up, but they were blocked. In the UK, the guidelines were rigidly enforced in some areas with patroling bobbies chasing people out of the water. One determined outdoor swimmer stopped because she couldn't stand the stares, the sense that onlookers were thinking, "Why should you get to swim when I can't?" A couple of months into the pandemic, swim memoirist Bonnie Tsui published an article in the *New York Times* entitled, "What I Miss Most Is Swimming." She wrote, "There's a poignancy to being a swimmer now, in that we're not able to do it just when we need it most.... Swimming is an antidote for the existential anxiety from which I suffer."

I was always disdainful of those single-lane lap pools and the so-called "endless pool," a jet resistance you swim against, basically going nowhere, endlessly! But with the shutdown of conventional pools, swimmers were buying them or, more commonly, wishing they could afford to. Meanwhile, the open-water community in the UK refused to take the situation lying down. A flurry of posts sprouted on the OSS and other online sites about blow-up backyard pools. Yes, folks who proudly describe themselves as wild swimmers were ordering blue plastic inflatable pools on Amazon, setting them up in their backyards, tethering themselves to a stationary object and proceeding to swim in place. Swimmers who hate chlorinated pools were dumping chorine into their backyard pools so they wouldn't become germ-infested. They patted themselves on the back for making do, with cheery British pluck. And as pitiful as it all looked to me, I could totally understand. It's an addiction, this need to be in water. I even felt a bit guilty. They had postage-stamp-sized pools, and I had a Great Lake.

After the full-on lockdown eased up in early summer, outdoor pools in Toronto began to re-open but with restrictions. The city imposed strict limits on the number of people in the pool at any one time, and each swimmer was limited to forty-five minutes. Between shifts, the pools were cleared and surfaces sterilized. People found they had to wait in line, sometimes for hours, and often didn't even manage to get into the water. Lanes had to be booked ahead of time. Lockers were off-limits. Time in change rooms was minimized: Swimmers were encouraged to wear their suits to the pool and home again. Once they managed to get into the facility, some users found themselves singing the praises of the restrictions. "Forty people is nothing. You feel like you have the place to yourself. Maintaining distance is a breeze," Ian Brown wrote in the *Globe and Mail*. Still, in the middle of a summer heat wave, Toronto pools were operating at a quarter of their capacity, in a city that sits beside an enormous freshwater lake.

Now, I don't believe that the big concrete-and-chlorine tubs are going to disappear, nor do I think they should. But I look forward to the day when they're no longer the default option for getting into the water. Covid-19 changed the swimming universe. In the fall of 2020, indoor pools in Toronto were declared off-limits again, after re-opening in mid-July. And the various open-water and wild-swimming sites I follow on Facebook showed a huge jump in interest.

I found evidence of this in my own backyard. A neighbor who is a dedicated pool swimmer told me the lake was too cold for her, even in the summer, but the lockdown forced her hand. During the summer, she broke down and bought a neoprene suit. Off Ward's Beach, a line of buoys keeps boats out of the swimming area. We reckon they are a little more than 50 meters (164 feet) apart. Most days, I saw her doing her daily 1,500 meters (almost a mile) between the buoys. (Okay, so it *is* possible to swim lengths in a lake.)

The wild-swimming trend, which may have begun as a necessary adjustment to pandemic conditions, is taking hold worldwide, as more and more swimmers go for regular dips in open-air pools, lakes, and rivers. At one point, demand in the UK was so high that the Outdoor Swimming

Society was forced to take down its map of wild-swimming spots in an attempt to prevent overcrowding. Even colder weather, more challenging water temperatures, and the discomfort of wriggling into dry clothing in public failed to deter many converts. The National Open Water Coaching Association, which operates bookings for thirty open-water venues in England and Scotland, said the number of swimmers in October 2020 was up nearly 400 per cent year on year, after a 60 per cent rise in swimmers over the summer. The surge in outdoor swimming was a boon for watersports suppliers. Sales of swimsuits fell because of the closure of indoor pools, but cold-water swimming gear—wetsuits, dry robes, neoprene swimcaps—flew off the shelves.

Covid-19 introduced countless water lovers to the joys of open water, and many will never go back. As one convert wrote on an open-water swimming site, "Ya gotta love not having to book lanes at the pool."

CHAPTER 6

The Winter of the Log Ness Monster:
Diary of my cold-water year

Every day for 365 days —
a swim in Lake Ontario

**Island resident Kathleen McDonnell
completes self-imposed challenge**
CBC News · Posted: Apr 25, 2016

Winter didn't feel as mild for Kathleen McDonnell as it did for most Torontonians. Rain or shine, whether it was warm or if she was punching through hunks of ice with her fists, the Ward's Island resident went for a swim in Lake Ontario every day for the past year.

McDonnell took her 365th consecutive dip in the lake today.

"I do it because I enjoy it," she told CBC Radio's *Metro Morning.* "It makes me feel vigorous and young. As I get older it's one of those things I think really helps me manage life."

"But I'm not one of these people who want to climb a mountain, and I don't take many risks."

McDonnell goes in wearing a one-piece swimsuit, cap, goggles, and some scuba gloves. The water was about 8 C during one of her recent swims, and she stayed out for about 15 minutes.

McDonnell's lived on the island for about 30 years but grew up in Chicago where, she says, people spent much more time on the less developed lakeshore.

"Everybody went to the beach and everybody went in the lake," she recalls. "It was just part of what everybody did in the summer."

Previously, she would stop swimming in the lake in November but, last year, decided to push on through winter. On one of the colder days, McDonnell had to punch through sheets of ice to make her way. But, she says, she always put in her time, even if sometimes she was less than enthusiastic.

"There were days that were hard just because the weather was so miserable," she says. "If it was raining and windy all day I would just find a chunk of that day when I felt 'Okay, I can do this.'"

"I'm lucky to be in a place where I can get in the water whenever I want."

ANDY WARHOL ONCE said that everyone in the world would be famous for fifteen minutes, but I wasn't really looking for my fifteen minutes. Not for this.

In fact, I didn't tell anyone I was planning a consecutive 365-day swim in open water, in essence reviving the practice of the Psychrolute Society. Honestly, there was no plan. I just kind of fell into it: did my usual winter swimming thing and…kept going.

By early December 2015, I was still "dipping"—that's what I call it, rather than swimming. My routine hasn't changed. I put on my old, ratty blue tank suit; old, ratty-but-still-warm black down jacket from the nineties (Sundown label, Island vintage); old, ratty Island-logo blue tuque; neoprene socks; and old, ratty, slip-on (and yes, blue!) Crocs. If the wind and waves aren't too bad, I proceed to the far eastern end of Ward's Beach, tear off everything but the tank, tuque, and neoprene socks, and quickly walk into the waist-high water until I'm up to my neck, keeping my hands clasped as if in prayer—honestly, it's just the easiest way to keep them out of the water. I make random noises, talk to myself, usually sing a non-sense song or made-up melody as I prance around, head and hands above water, for at least three minutes (yes, I count to sixty three times). While in the water, I survey the length of the beach to see if there are any people around, especially if they're coming anywhere near me. I hate that. I don't want to worry about what they're thinking, wondering whether I'm a crazy, old lady or a person in distress. If it's too windy on the beach, I opt instead for a spot on the city-side, a little stretch of beach just west of the Eastern Gap, where it's sheltered and no one sees me (well, hardly ever).

When it's time to come out, I throw on everything I took off, starting with the down jacket, and head back to the other end of the beach, up the path to Lakeshore Road. I've never actually timed it, but the walk back to my house takes about five or six minutes. The only part of me that really feels cold is my toes. I take a nice, hot bath, during the early moments of which I feel a shimmer of cold coming off my back into the water, like my body is cooling down the hot water. I feel enlivened, shaken out of my passivity, negativity, and laziness.

The winters of 2013–2014 and 2014–2015 were fiercely cold, with thick ice covering Toronto harbor (which was, among other things, a huge disruption to our Island ferry service). The previous few seasons had been milder—in fact, the harbor was nearly ice-free through most winters of the early twenty-first century, which looked like it was becoming the new normal. So it wasn't surprising to see the weather pattern shift again in late 2015. November and December were very mild, sometimes with daytime temperatures in the double digits. With the appearance of what meteorologists called an extreme El Niño, it appeared more likely that a mild winter was in store, reducing the odds that ice build-up would prevent access to open water. I realized this was the year to aim for a 365-day swim but I decided to make my decision on a day-by-day basis.

I had always followed certain parameters as winter arrived: no swimming in sub-zero temperatures; in big wind and waves; or with no sun. In January 2016, things became much more winter-like. Daytime temperatures were often below 0 C (32 F), and by mid-month spectacular skating ice had formed in the lagoons. I began to break all my rules. Every day I walked to the far eastern end of Ward's Beach, where I could find a bit of shelter from the wind, and waded quickly into water that was at least waist-high. If there were big waves, I didn't try to swim, just gamboled around in the water. Every morning, I checked the hourly forecast to see when it was most likely to be sunny, and I said thank you if the sun was out when I entered and, especially, came out of the water. I went in regardless, for anywhere from two to five minutes, depending on conditions, fully immersed up to my neck, wearing my sleeveless neoprene shortie, socks, and gloves.

I decided to follow the lead of Roger Deakins and started keeping my own "waterlog."

JANUARY 21, 2016

There was a fierce wind on the beach. Overall I felt fine when I emerged from the water, except for my hands. I had a terrible time getting my clothes back on. I finally managed to get dressed and set off, but my hands stayed hard as rocks all the way back to my house. It freaked me out. It's a hard lesson I have to keep relearning: You gotta take special care with your hands. How far along on the evolutionary scale would we humans have come without them?

Like an incident a few weeks earlier, I found myself wrestling with a stronger undertow than Lake Ontario usually serves up, and I realized I was more vulnerable to the elements than I'd thought. I resolved to alter my swim habits, so as not to get myself into that kind of situation again, but I wasn't sure exactly how I was going to avoid it.

In the winter, windchill is almost always a factor on Ward's Beach. For a day or so, the wind was a bit calmer, but on the way home I realized my neoprene gloves had fallen out of my jacket pocket. I retraced my steps and found one, but not the other. *Oh well*, I thought, *I'll have to buy a new pair.* They didn't really keep my hands warm anyway. Maybe it was time to see if there were better neoprene gloves on the market. The next day, I invested in a pair of scuba diving gloves. They cost twice as much as my old gloves, and they were a bitch to pull on and off, but they were way thicker neoprene and much tighter, so my hands were far better insulated. When I got out of the water I could function fine and dress quickly: no rock-hard, clumsy fingers. Another winter swimming obstacle overcome.

Ward's Beach is about 350 meters long (about a quarter mile). At the far eastern end, there's a wall of large rocks and demolition scrap the city deposited decades ago as a breakwater to prevent erosion of the beach, which had been disappearing fast. One of our island neighbors, Tyler, is an arborist who makes furniture and other structures from his trimmed cuts. A few years ago, he felled a dying tree and gouged it out, creating a dugout canoe. At one end, he carved a dragon head, and rigged it so the creature could be made to breathe fire when gasoline was shot through some tubing and lit, at the opening of its huge, gaping maw. The Log Ness Monster, as Tyler and his friends christened the creature, didn't have a long career as a fire-breather because it encountered mechanical failure after a few demonstrations. Log Ness Monster was abandoned on Ward's Beach near the breakwater, gradually filling with sand so that little more than its craning neck was visible.

Most days, at the far end of the beach, there was just me, a few wintering-over ducks, the occasional mute swan, and the Log Ness Monster, whose head provided a handy coat rack for my jacket, and whose neck served as a railing for me to grab as I stepped across slippery sheets of ice on my way into the water.

JANUARY 22, 2016

Another fairly calm day on the beach. No need to take the water temperature. There was a thin skin of sheet ice a few yards out from shore. I've become so well acquainted with the lake through these winter swims. Noticed that though the water is just cold enough for ice to form, it rarely stays for very long because it's broken by the movement of the water—sometimes waves, even gentle ripples, as happened today.

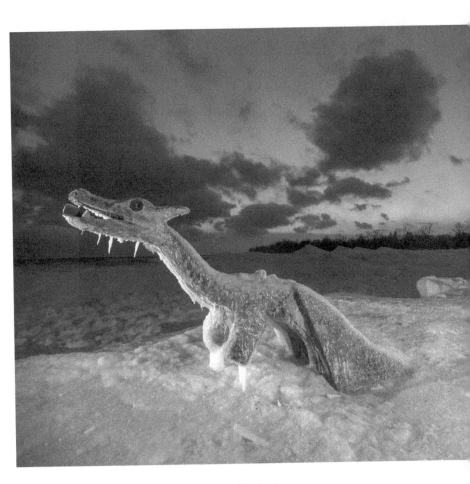

"The Log Ness Monster encased in ice."
Photo by Sean Tamblyn.

JANUARY 26, 2016

A lovely swim. No problem—only light wind and near 0 C (32 F) temperatures. I stayed in for four or five minutes, which I counted, as reluctant as I am to quantify this endeavor. The cold-water swimmers on Facebook are tenacious in reporting how much time they spend in the water, how far they swim and of course, stress they only wear a standard swimsuit (the Brits call it a swimming costume), with no gloves, a regular cap, etc. Although I want to resist getting into a competition with these hardcores, I decided to try a regular tank suit this week, when the air temperature is above zero.

I'd bought a big suit—a full wetsuit—on my last birthday, thinking it would encourage me to go colder in my 365 attempt. But I also realized how much it totally insulated me—*cut me off*—from the water. It was too heavy and bulky, felt like a suit of armor. I'd assumed there was no way I could swim through a Lake Ontario winter without one, but that hasn't turned out to be the case at all. My sleeveless shortie is just fine. In fact, I hated the full wetsuit.

So what I've learned is: I don't need it. I can handle the cold water just fine.

FEBRUARY 6, 2016

I've been staying in the water consistently for three to five minutes, swimming a short distance when I can, and just bobbing around when it's too rough. The water temp has been hovering around freezing, and I've continued to be amazed at how easy it has been—how comfortable, yes!—in water that cold, as long as I protect my hands. If I do the winter swim event next month in Vermont, the rules say I'll have to do it without gloves, which shouldn't be a problem with Alec, my spouse, there to wrap me up and help me get dressed afterwards.

I'm also getting less hung up on being seen when I swim. I realize it's a small price to pay for doing something so out of the ordinary. It's *outdoor* swimming after all. There are other people on the beach too. Why I have such a resistance to being *seen*, I have no idea. Perhaps it's from growing up in my family, my mother in particular: Don't stand out. Don't call attention to yourself.

FEBRUARY 16, 2016

Real winter has arrived and I knew these few days would be the watershed moment (another lame pun) for my 365 streak. Three days ago, when the high temperature was -17 C (1 F), I thought it would be the most challenging; but the bitter cold turned out to be no big deal. The western end of Ward's Beach was sheltered enough to avoid wind-chill. There were waves one day, but the lake has been mostly calm, and I swam for two or three minutes in my shortie, with spotters Alec and Ty on shore, ready to help me get dressed fast.

Yesterday was tricky. It has been fun to break through thin skins of ice, but they were too thick, covering the length of Ward's Beach. In other words, there was no open water to be had at the Ward's end of the island. People wanted to go for a skate. I'd skated and swum (well, plunged) on the same day a few times before. For me, skating is another way of communing with the water, the only thing that gives me the same exhilaration as cold-water swimming. In or on the water, that's the thing.

So, with a whole crew of spotters this time (Alec, Liz, Rick), we biked to Centre Island, where there was a nice pool of open water next to the Pier. Full wetsuit this time, because I needed to keep warm on the bike ride back to Ward's. After my swim, the crew took off to skate on Long Pond, and I rode home.

FEBRUARY 25, 2016

Today, a new wrinkle: snow, lots of it, along with a much milder air temp (around 0 C or 32 F). I woke up and wondered, would today be the deal breaker? Would I be forced to interrupt my streak? But no. At the western end of Ward's Beach, where thick ice had covered the shoreline only the day before, there was a calm pool of open water, with a few bobbing slabs of ice. The force was with me.

MARCH 1, 2016

You'd think the toughest challenge of a 365-day winter swim would have been a couple of weeks ago, when the air temp topped out at -17 C (1 F). But no, not with the sunshine and calm waters, not by a long shot. Today was a much tougher test—gray sky, snow on the ground, -7 C (19 F), fierce wind. I decided the wind is the true enemy of the cold-water swimmer. I knew this was going to be one of those let's-get-this-over-with swims. Fun didn't enter into the equation. The past few wintry days I went to my new spot, a tiny, sheltered beach just off First Street (sorry, Log Ness, hope you missed me!) to the east of what islanders call the cove. Threw off my down jacket and fleece pants, walked in the water, dunked up to my neck, counted to 120, walked out. Mission accomplished.

MARCH 2, 2016

I'd been hearing about an event called the Winter Swimming Festival in northern Vermont, where organizers cut a two-lane, 25-meter (82-foot) "pool" out of the ice in Lake Memphremagog, a glacial lake that straddles the border with Quebec. The festival was only in its second year, and I was keen to go; but preparing for the trip, I had to figure out how to continue my streak. I was within shot of 365. All swims to that point had been on my home ground Lake Ontario. I decided my streak would be legitimate as long as I did an outdoor swim of some kind.

That would be no problem when we got to Lake Memphremagog. En route was the issue. We were traveling by train to Montreal, and driving a rental car east to northern Vermont the next day. Outdoor swimming is a challenge in Montreal, even in the summer. The city sits on the magnificent St. Lawrence River, but has one artificially created beach in Parc Jean-Drapeau, accessible by subway. Was it iced-over? Probably, given that Montreal is colder than Toronto. I googled every which way I could think of. There was a rowing channel in the park. Was it open? Would I be in trouble if I tried to go in? The pickings were slim and there were complications. Time was getting short.

I shifted focus: what about an outdoor pool? My bias, overwhelmingly, was for natural bodies of water, but I needed to fill a one-day gap. I decided it wouldn't invalidate my streak so long as it was outdoors. A hotel at Place Bonaventure had a rooftop pool—open all year!—a stone's-throw from the train station with a single-day fee. I sent a special request to see whether I could have access for an afternoon, thought if I gave them a pitch about my open-water streak maybe they'd take pity on me, do it for public spiritedness, maybe even a bit of publicity. Days went by. No answer. We were due to leave for Montreal. It was beginning to look like there was only one way to be sure I could get in an outdoor swim: Book a room at the Hotel Bonaventure. I found a deal on Expedia for a minimum two-night stay, $90 a night. Quite a chunk of change for a dip in a pool.

MARCH 3, 2016

Some new wrinkles in preparation for the Memphremagog swim: Today I swam with bare feet, no booties. The past few days, I'd been swimming without my neoprene gloves. And once I went in a regular tank suit, instead of my neoprene shortie. The latter was easy. I hardly felt any difference (though it certainly would have mattered if I'd tried to stay in longer than the three minutes I did). But I'd gotten accustomed to protecting my hands and feet. Going in with them bare, I felt a bit of cold shock, not only in the extremities themselves, but in my legs and arms. Hands are the real killer. Actual pain added to my anxiety that my hands were going to be damaged. But it'll be English Channel rules in Vermont. No neoprene allowed. I'll have to go barehanded.

MARCH 4, 2016

At the Hotel Bonaventure. As hotel pools go, this one's fairly large, more than two strokes long. I had it all to myself. (Why was that, do you suppose?) Snowdrifts around the pool. Water was too warm, but brisk air made up for it. It was -3 C (26.6 F) out, but sunny. For a pool swim, it was more than adequate.

MARCH 5, 2016 (VERMONT)

Waiting to swim 25-meter freestyle. Unaccountably anxious. Writing to calm myself. Not worried about the water temp, more that it's an unfamiliar situation. Post swim #1: finally calming down. I got so scattered before the swim—trying to keep track of my stuff; what I had to wear onto the ice; wondering when my turn would come up—that I was barely present for the swim itself. It went by too fast. Barely had time to feel the cold water. No problem at all with my hands. I could easily have stayed in longer. I *wanted* to stay in longer.

Interesting, I feel my good mood has returned. After two days of no cold-water immersion following days and days of consecutive cold-water swims, I could feel my mood darkening—not hugely, not to depression level, but it felt like I'd become dependent, addicted to the daily experience. The warm-water pool, even though it was out-doors, just didn't cut it. I was going through withdrawal.

The festival was a strictly no-wetsuit event and had the feel of a summer camp but in below-zero temperatures. Fleshy women abounded! Men too, but it was notable that many of the women were, well, overweight by existing social standards because (no surprise) certain bodies—ones with more fat—are better equipped to handle the cold. Notice I didn't say health standards. These heavy women (I include myself) were, to all appearances, as healthy as horses. The exceptions were the competitive swimmers, who are all, male and female, long and lean and muscu-lar. They shot through the water like arrows. At the awards dinner, the same trio of lithe, skinny women claimed first, second and third in various events. That's why they were there: to win, to place. But I'm quite certain that if these races were longer distances, we fleshy types would have lasted a lot longer in the sub-zero water. Like my old swim-ming mentor Klaus said, "We have padding."

The concept of racing through water is so completely foreign to me, so little to do with why I swim, something that became clearer than ever to me at Lake Memphremagog. As I entered the water for the second "race," 50 meters (164 feet), I told myself not to worry about keeping up, to swim in my usual way and enjoy myself. I was my slow-as-molasses self, but managed to remind myself to relax enough to *feel* the water, to experience and even luxuriate in the coldness. That made it more satisfying than the over-before-it-started experience of the 25-meter. The swimmer in the other lane finished way ahead of me, of course, but I let myself be more present during the swim. (Yeah, I realize how Zen that sounds, don't hate me.) Meanwhile, on the sidelines, I could sense some people were concerned that I was having difficulty, that I was in the water "too long." They cheered—in relief, mostly—when I finished, and told me I had done really well. It was the kind of compliment the hard-core, confident ones, the racers, give novices or children. A for effort. I knew their support was genuine and appreciated it. What they did not know was that I (and I suspect most cold-water enthusiasts) bring a profoundly different attitude to the activity. Not only do I not care about winning or placing, I actively dislike the racing mindset because swimming fast counters the enjoyment of swimming in the cold. Racers want to get out of the water as quickly as possible. Me, I want to stay in as long as I (safely and comfortably) can.

So, in some ways my third swim, though shorter than I would have chosen, was the most satisfying. I requested an extra out-of-competition swim on Sunday, explaining that I wanted to keep my 365 streak going. Phil, the organizer, very graciously let me slip into the final heat of the 25-meter butterfly, since one of the lanes was open. He said to swim as long as I wanted, but I didn't want to overstay my welcome and did only one length.

MARCH 11, 2016

I don't remember how long I've been having swimming dreams, but they occur regularly. Occasionally they're about enjoyment (sometimes near-ecstatic) of being in water, but most have an element of danger or, most frequently, denial of water. I can see it, but can't quite get to it. The water is thick, slushy ice, but I plough through it. This one's in the latter category:

"I won't let anything keep me out of the water."

On a beach, not Ward's, looks much more like Touhy Ave, from my childhood. It's still water, there are patches of snow and ice. I'm determined to swim, but the beach has changed, now fortified by a huge wall jutting out into the water. On the other side of the beach, there's a chain-link fence blocking the way to the adjoining beach to the south. This seriously impedes access to the water. Even the small patch of shoreline is blocked by a highway. There's no way to get in or out. It certainly looks like someone is trying to prevent swimming here.

But I won't let anything keep me out of the water. Through the chain-link fence I can see open water and a man lifting the bottom of the fence and slipping underneath it. I do the same, though now I'm worried that I may get caught doing something forbidden. There's still a lot of snow and ice on the shoreline, but at least no wall preventing me from getting into the water. Before I do, the dream ends.

MARCH 17, 2016: ST. PATRICK'S DAY

Sláinte!

One quality this cold-water swimming promotes is adaptation. Humans—at least we humans in the modern, developed world—aren't called upon to *adapt* much anymore. So much is under (or we attempt to *put* it under) our control that we've succeeded in forcing the world to adapt to us and our desires. Evolution is the opposite: Adapt or be eliminated! Just to give an example in a swimming context: You go to a pool, and the water temp is always controlled, "adapted" to a standard that suits the majority. There are no waves, winds, cold air temps to deal with because you're indoors. It's pretty much true for outdoor pools too. Swimming outdoors, in a natural body of water, you have to accept and adapt to the existing conditions, which change every time you go. You don't have a say in the matter. Things are what they are. You deal with it. If the water is cold, well, adapt or walk away. If the water is choppy or rough, accept and go in—or not, if it's just too dangerous. The water is in charge, not you.

I'm convinced that part of the extreme pleasure, the *high* of swimming in cold water, comes from this necessity to adapt, to persevere and prevail against all odds. There's a particular joy that surfaces when the conditions are—for this person, at this moment—*just right*: The sun is out, the water is flat, the air is calm, and the temperature (water or air) is cold and bracing, and you feel alive. You didn't manage this: It's a gift. You may have asked for it, wished for it, hoped for it, but you knew damned well it wasn't under your control. So you are grateful and enjoy it. Sometimes, on a cloudy day the sun comes out just as I'm entering the water (it's probably my wishful thinking, but it really does seem to happen often), and I say "thank you."

I seem to be saying that the joy of an activity like swimming is inversely proportional to the control one can exert over it. The same is true of wild skating. The thickness of the ice, the smooth, glide-able surface—it's a gift that Mother Nature decides to bestow, or not, whenever it suits her.

I have to admit, I don't think my adaptability to open-water swimming has carried over to the rest of my life in a significant way. I'm still a control freak.

APRIL 5, 2016:
THE RETURN OF THE POLAR VORTEX

After the cold snap in March, I thought I was home free for my 365. Little did I know that not only was winter not done with us, she was bringing a polar vortex for good measure. I don't think a scientific dissertation on this phenomenon is necessary or warranted. It just means that, more than two weeks after the supposed beginning of spring, it is effing cold; cold enough to numb my hands when I emerge from the water and take off my neoprene gloves, but not cold enough (for long enough) to allow ice to form on Ward's Beach, which has been covered in a couple inches of snow. I thought this early-April stretch would be a piece of cake. Hah! Today, as I pulled on my shortie, I thought to myself that I'm fed up with swimming in this shitty weather.

APRIL 14, 2016

For years people have asked me, "How can you swim in that water? It's polluted!" As though Lake Ontario is nothing but a cesspool. I call that the yuck factor. The fear factor also kicks in when the water is dark. For some people it's almost a phobia. Is it the loss of control ("You can't see the bottom!"), the terror of what might be lurking down there, even the memory of floating in the dark, enclosed womb?

I don't know what they're talking about: Fear of water is foreign to my consciousness. Water always beckons, never frightens me. Sure, there are times when conditions are scary and I have to tell myself not to succumb to the desire to plunge in. That stems from knowledge. It shows *respect* for what water can do. But the idea of water being scary in and of itself? To me that's unthinkable.

And lastly, there's the cold factor: "Oooh, how can you? It makes me shiver just to *think* about going in that water," or "I could never do it...." The tensing up, the shrinking back from the very idea of cold water. Where does that come from? Biology? Evolution? It is learned and can be unlearned. Again, something that feels so normal, so not-a-big-deal to me elicits such intense feelings of avoidance in so many people. I feel like I am another sort of creature altogether—human, but somehow completely at home in the water, with a constant drive to be in the water, on it (ice), or near it.

APRIL 25, 2016

This morning, I headed to Ward's Beach and plunged into the water for swim #365, then told a few friends, including Liz, who called a radio show to tell them about my streak. Okay, fine. It felt like no big deal, but it seemed to be a big deal to the people around me. Something told me my so-what attitude was, well, unhealthy? Dismissive of self? Why didn't I want to make a big deal of pulling off something that few other people have?

Partly it was because I thought my "achievement" was too easy. I didn't have to push myself. I *wanted* to do it. It gave a shape to every day, and I'm moving into the time of life where that's important; having something concrete to *do* every fucking day, so old age, which is basically filling in the time until the end, has a structure, a purpose. Yes, I realize that's awfully flippant, but at the most basic level it's true. We're all filling in time, but sometimes we're more aware of it than others. And no. I don't really believe I've reached old age. I feel like I'm about, oh, 35.

The other part of the dismissal is the central conundrum of my life: a craving to be *seen*, to be acknowledged, honored, is combined with a desire to be *invisible*. And, now that I'm older and more settled in my ways, I realize how demanding, invasive, and exhausting it can be to be recognized, honored, *famous*. When I was in high school my ambition was to be on the cover of *Time* magazine! I'm actually kind of glad I've avoided all that. And yet, I still want it. I guess on my own terms—maybe myself not visible, just my writing? By her written words ye shall know her? A question has been gnawing at me lately (in line with the philosophy that we create our own reality, which I think is mostly, but not completely, bullshit): Am I unknown, invisible because I chose to be?

MAY 19, 2016

It finally happened. I was on the beach, sitting with my back against the big log, taking in the modest warmth of the sun and psyching myself up to brave the stiff wind coming from the west. Two women wearing cycling helmets came down the path. One walked to the shore, took off her biking glove and felt the water. (I've seen beach visitors doing this quite a bit lately.) The other came over and asked me how the water was. I started to answer when she broke in, "Are you the lady who swims all year in the lake?"

"Yep, that's me," I said.

"I heard you on the radio."

We had a nice chat, exchanged glad-to-meet-yous, etc. They went back up the path, and I decided it was time to get my ass in the water. My fifteen minutes of fame are (not quite) over.

MAY 25, 2016

Since my #365 swim, I've had more questions than usual about hypothermia, i.e., don't I get hypothermic going into such cold water? The answer, of course, is no—as I try to explain how I enter the water calmly, how I've trained myself to cope, how a lot of it is mental, and so on, their eyes usually glaze over after a few phrases. They're just not that interested, I think, because it doesn't sound like anything they could or would want to do. Some weird preoccupation from a foreign universe. In the real world, no one *likes* cold water, and any sensible person avoids contact with it. Seeing their lack of interest, I usually don't go on to my next point, that I have only experienced hypothermia once in my life, and it was at an indoor pool.

It was at a Toronto hotel pool near the ferry docks where I used to maintain a membership before I went full-bore open water. The pool had been drained for maintenance and refilled, and the attendant said it hadn't yet warmed up to swimming temperature. Oh, I'll bet it has for me, I thought, and asked if I could go for a quick swim anyway.

I don't know what the water temp actually was, but as I slowly entered the shallow end, I was quite sure it wasn't as cold as some of my Lake Ontario swims. I swam a few lengths without discomfort. After a few minutes, though, I could feel something was different about the water. It just wasn't the same as a natural body of water. It felt somehow not...alive. Yes, I know it was chemically the same as the lake—in fact, most assuredly "cleaner" with the addition of chlorine. But it just didn't feel right. I knew I had to get out of the pool. Immediately.

On the pool deck, I didn't feel particularly cold, I wasn't shivering at all. But I was disoriented. It was fairly quiet in the pool area (only the attendant was with me) but every sound—the water, the attendant's voice as he spoke into the phone—reverberated in my head like an echo. Things around me had a hallucinatory quality. I just wasn't right in the head, but I couldn't let the pool attendant know: pride. I hoped I was steady enough to walk to the change room. Carefully, I made my way to the shower stall where I turned on the hot water almost full blast and let it pour over me for I don't know how many minutes till gradually I felt my normal consciousness returning. I still hadn't shivered, even slightly, but I knew that what I had experienced was a sudden onset of hypothermia. I, who swam regularly and comfortably in 10 C (50 C) water, and since then have increased my tolerance even further. It's still a mystery why it happened in water temp that posed no problem for me in the lake. Call me a flake, I continue to believe it had something to do with the absence of some quality of *vitality* in the chemically treated pool. In years of swimming, this was my one and only experience of cold-water-induced hypothermia, and I'm glad I had it.

So this is how it comes on: pouncing quickly, barely noticed. So this is what it does to your mental state, your judgment. Good to know. Good to know.

JUNE 17, 2016:
BE CAREFUL WHAT YOU WISH FOR

I'd been going to regular Sacred Harp singings in Toronto for several years, but had never made the trek to Camp Fasola (yes, it's really called that) in Alabama. My singing buddy Frank had been encouraging me to go, and said there was room for me in his car, but I had a hard time making the decision. I, who can't stand the heat, head to Alabama in June? In the week leading up to the trip, I checked the weather forecast and was dismayed to see an unbroken stretch of days in the 90s (I could use Celsius but this was the USA, and "in the 30s" just doesn't suggest the same wallop of debilitating heat). But there was a pool and a small lake on the grounds where the camp was being held. I figured if I could submerge myself in water at least once a day, I could bear the heat.

We set off from Toronto for two long days of driving. Toward the end of the second day, I was desperate to get into water and I learned from Google, to my surprise, that Alabama had an abundance of swimming holes and reservoirs. I scoped out one at a spot called Little River Canyon, just off the highway. It had a waterfall! A plunge into some cool, rushing water? I was *there*. I boldly talked my companions into making the stop, which turned out to be a longer, more out-of-the-way drive than I'd expected. The group was eager to arrive at camp and get settled in. The prospect of an unscheduled stop led to some grumbling, mostly unspoken, but I could feel it in the air—until we got to the entrance to the conservation area, and someone noticed a historical plaque at the side of the road. It was a Trail of Tears marker, about a band of 1,103 Cherokee who voluntarily emigrated from their homeland in Tennessee in 1838. Led by their own Indigenous leadership, they planned to continue living as a free Nation in Oklahoma, governed by their own laws and constitution. That dream went unrealized, of course, and many suffered the same fate as other Indigenous nations on the Trail of Tears. We were all moved to be standing in the place those Cherokee had passed through more than a century earlier.

Little River Falls turned out to be pretty, a zone of smooth rock shelves and small boulders, but without much water. Mostly it only came up as far as my waist. By itself that wasn't a problem. I could squat and even swim around a bit, but it was warm. Pea-soup warm. Warmer than I thought fast-moving water over rocks could ever be. I got wet, but refreshing? Uh, no.

I was thrilled to discover, on arrival at camp, that I'd been assigned to a cabin overlooking the lake. Did I say lake? It turned out to be more like a pond. I made my way down the side of a small hill with brambles and patches of dry grass to a spot where I could walk into the water. It was a muddy, reddish-clay bottom and I sank in up to my knees as soon as I waded in. I lunged forward to keep from sinking further into the clay. Warm water. Too warm. Almost bathtub warm. Other than in some hot springs a few years earlier, I had never encountered such warm temperatures in an outdoor body of water. About ten or twelve inches further in, the water temperature changed abruptly, becoming markedly cooler. I plunged below the surface several times to enjoy the coolness, and was reluctant to venture into the tepid water up top. But I got wet. I even swam a little.

The next day I had a pool swim. Nothing to say about it, really. Too warm, but that was to be expected. Then I went to the pond again. This time the water was even warmer, and the zone of cooler water underneath had pretty much disappeared.

I couldn't wait to get home to my beloved Lake Ontario. No more of this warm-as-pea-soup nonsense. I was dying to cool off. I got back to the island and headed to the beach. As soon as I put one foot in the water, it was clear that conditions were different from when I'd left a week earlier. Something had occurred, an event I've come to think of as the June Flip, when the lake, having begun to warm up in the few hot days of late May, takes a 180-degree turn. I submerged myself. Whoa! It was frigid (not a word I use often in regards to water). Frigid enough to numb my fingers. Frigid enough that it hurt to put my face in. Frigid the way it had been back in April and early May.

The next day I took my plastic pool thermometer down to the beach. When I put my foot in the water, it felt ever so slightly warmer than the day before. I stuck in the thermometer and held it under for several seconds, then brought it back up. 12 C (54 F). I'd said I wanted to cool off. Be careful what you wish for.

JUNE 5, 2016

When I first moved to Toronto Island, lots of people went to the beach but very few went in the water. It was a—not unreasonable—fear of pollution, given the city's practice of allowing untreated sewage to spill into the lake during heavy storms. Though I doubt there was much water-quality testing of Chicago's beaches back in the day and that didn't deter beach-goers in the least. In the case of Toronto, I think it was a lack of swimming culture that made locals shun the water. In contrast to Chicago, with

its near-unbroken string of beaches along the city's eastern edge, Toronto's waterfront was heavily industrialized
with few beaches or even inviting spots to be near the water.
When I started swimming regularly in the lake, I heard a
lot of comments and questions along the lines of, "You
couldn't pay me to swim in that cesspool," and "Don't you
get sick?" Often, I was treated to neighbors' accounts of
the severe illnesses they suffered as a result (they were quite
convinced) of swimming in the lake. I assured them that,
no, I had never been sick after being in the lake, jokingly
adding that after a lifetime of swimming in the Great Lakes,
I must have developed antibodies to all the pollutants.

But I didn't really think that at all. I thought my experience was normal, that the people who blamed the lake
for their illnesses were wrong, that they were driven by a
belief, a widespread fear and loathing about water that I
didn't share—that, in fact, mystified me. The sight of water,
far from repelling me or making me wary, draws me in. I
have never (well, almost never) met a natural body of water
that I didn't long to plunge into. Still, I played along with
my interrogators' views on the unfitness of natural water:
"Well, I haven't sprouted a second head yet," I'd say jocularly.
Occasionally, I'd try reason and logic, pointing out that if
the water's polluted, it might make a person sick right away
with an earache or sick stomach. But the effects of most
toxic chemicals can linger for a couple of decades, at which
point you learn you've got cancer. The turning away from
water runs deep. Take pollutants in the air that damage
your lungs and cause chronic illness. Sure, breathing isn't

a conscious choice, unlike the act of submerging oneself in water, but no one ever says, "You couldn't pay me enough to breathe that air." Though, maybe they should.

SEPTEMBER 16, 2016

In the ongoing quest to understand my water addiction, I often ponder, *Why?* Why do I have this urgent desire, this primal need to plunge into any body of water I encounter? What is it that separates people like me, the swimmers-at-all-costs, from those who are indifferent, turned off, or even frightened of being in water?

Today, on Ward's Beach a woman came with two dogs on leashes, both small and curly-haired—they were like canine twins! Cockapoos perhaps? (I'm not much for dog identification, especially not these latter-day designer breeds. My knowledge stops at Labs and German Shepherds.) There was one striking difference between them. One was pulling on the leash full force, its head stretched forward, eager (no, desperate) to get into the water. The other trotted along next to the woman. When they reached the shoreline, the first dog took a full-body plunge while the other lolled around in the sand, not the least bit interested in following her twin into the water. Here was a textbook demonstration of my question: What could explain the difference between these two almost identical individuals, one craving water and the other not? Another woman sitting on a blanket near the shore was also struck by the dogs' behavior, and commented to the owner. "Yes, that one loves the water," she said with a shrug.

Clearly she was familiar with the dogs' different responses, but not much interested in the mystery.

NOVEMBER 9, 2016

After a quick morning dip, I went to the airport and flew to New York City to meet up with my nieces, Caitlin and Emily. They'd both worked on Hillary Clinton's campaign, and we all went to the Javits Center to celebrate the historic election of the first female president of the United States. We know how that turned out. The day after the election, all I wanted to do was get in the water: real water, open water, wild water. Caitlin and I decided to go to Coney Island. I took the F train from 23rd Street station, got off at the New York Aquarium, walked through the parking lot to the boardwalk, and met up with her there. We walked down the ramp to the long, wide beach, the funhouse buildings on our right, and headed toward the shore. The air was mild, the water still not too cold, certainly not for us. There were a few people on the beach, but far off in the distance. Caitlin hadn't brought a swimsuit, and I figured what the hell. We both stripped and went in naked.

We took phone photos of each other in the water, our arms raised in tribute to Hillary. In the photos we look almost triumphant, which isn't a bad thing, though it certainly wasn't how we felt. The incongruity of it reminded me of Nixon leaving the White House after his resignation, suddenly, awkwardly throwing up his arms in a triumphal gesture completely at odds with the occasion.

On the bus to LaGuardia the next day, I listened to the

bus driver sing, "Big girls, they don't cry-yi-yi!" at the top of his lungs, and felt my melancholy lift a bit. Who could stay sad in the presence of such unabashed exuberance? After a while, he took a break from singing and got into a conversation with a man in a nearby seat, apparently a co-worker. "So I guess this means you've turned Republican?" the other man asked. "No way, man!" the driver replied. "I'm still a Democrat. I've still got my card. I mean, I wasn't all that crazy about voting for Trump," he went on. "I just couldn't bring myself to vote for Hillary. You can't trust her. There's something...*off* about her. She has cold eyes."

NOVEMBER 19, 2016

Back in Toronto, still reeling from the shock of Clinton's loss, I took the GO Train to Oakville for the Great Lakes Trust twenty-four-hour relay swim. They really wanted me to come—my cold-water exploits made me a minor celebrity in this crowd. The idea had been for participants to swim to a buoy about 750 meters (almost a half-mile) out and back, in about twenty minutes. I was glad to hear the plan had changed to "go out to where it's deep enough, and swim along the shore for as long (or as short) a time as you want," because 1,500 meters would take me more like forty minutes. No way I wanted to spend that long in 8 C (46 F) water.

It was sunny and quite calm at Coronation Park Beach, the best conditions for a cold-water swim. I walked out calmly to where the water was waist-high, submerged to my shoulders a few times, then slid into the water and commenced a nice, easy stroke. I kept my face underwater right from the start, which I usually don't do in water that cold, but it didn't make my face hurt.

After a couple of back-and-forths, accompanied by a kayaker named John, I started counting strokes as a way of keeping track of time. Folks on shore were to signal John at the ten-minute mark, and I wanted a sense of how close I was to that goal. I estimated I'd been in the water about six or seven minutes when I saw John gesturing to me. I lifted my head to ask, "How long?"

"Ten minutes," he said. I had no problem deciding to keep going, and asked him to let me know when I'd hit the fifteen-minute mark. I still felt relaxed, the water felt fine on my skin. I thought of Hillary, her grit and toughness. When John called out "Fifteen!" I paused for a moment and looked at the people gathered on the shore. Another on-the-spot decision.

I lifted my arms, like I had at Coney Island, and called out, "I'm going for twenty!" A cheer went up on shore.

I resumed swimming with the same calm, deliberate strokes. I still felt fine. Until, at about seventeen or eighteen minutes, I didn't feel fine anymore. My hands started to hurt, which I've learned is the beginning of feeling not-right, distressed. And there was something else—a brain thing, a feeling that "I shouldn't be here." In retrospect, I realize it was similar to the feeling I had when I became hypothermic in the pool: "This isn't right." But I knew I still had my faculties, that John was behind me in the kayak, and there were people watching out for me on the shore. A warming tent was waiting for me there. I could go for another minute or two. And I did.

When I poked my head up, John nodded that I'd hit the twenty-minute mark, though I honestly wondered whether he was fudging the time so I'd feel okay about quitting. By then, the I-have-to-get-out-of-here brain message was very strong and getting a bit scary. I swam toward shore, stood up in the shallows, and walked out of the water, only slightly staggering, to warm applause. I was a bit brain-addled when I got to the warming tent. I kept looking around for my big, red down jacket, which wasn't with the rest of my stuff. Slurring my syllables, I asked one of the organizers to retrieve it, which he did. Inside the tent I found it hard to concentrate on the simple task of changing into dry clothes, especially since my hands were numb and useless. Gradually, feeling came back into them, and I managed to fasten the snaps on the down jacket to make myself presentable enough to emerge from the tent.

By then, another swimmer was in the water and the crowd's focus had moved on, which was fine with me. I sat on the sand and watched the swimmer go back and forth a few meters out from shore, as I had minutes before. It was then that the shivering started, so strongly it made my right leg jerk independently. It kept on like that for at least five minutes. It was my first real experience of afterdrop.

Several spectators came over to congratulate me. One even commented on how relaxed I looked, almost contemplative, how "lovely" my stroke was. Now *that* was a first for me.

NOVEMBER 23, 2016

Hard to keep swimming lately, though it's been more cold-plunge than actual swimming. Gray sky, cold, damp winds. Went to the far end of Ward's Beach, home of the Log Ness Monster, with more in mind than a plunge. A guy appeared at the other end of the beach with four dogs—big, energetic dogs, a couple of which started chasing after me. I didn't react, didn't engage, just wanted them to ignore me and let me swim in peace. The guy called them back, I arrived at the breakwater and hoped they'd leave the beach soon. They were still yapping and running around, but far enough that I figured they wouldn't pay me any mind. I took off my big, black, down jacket and pants, put on my thick scuba gloves and glided into the water. It was calm, at least. I was comfortable enough, and started my strokes.

Halfway along the rocks, I looked up and saw a large, white bird perched atop the breakwater, gazing down at me. A snowy owl, looking unperturbed by my presence. Because I was excited, I wanted to acknowledge it without causing upset, so I spoke in a low, friendly tone of voice that I've used in other wildlife encounters. "Well, look at you. Look. At. You." A gift, in a sense (though that sounds a bit too human-centric, a bit too all-about-me), more like a visitation for which I was grateful. I swam farther along the rocks, and the owl continued to perch and look around, unruffled. When I turned to swim back to shore, I saw the guy with the four dogs heading toward us, me and Snowy, and I was upset. I didn't want the dogs carrying on, barking at me in the water. Even though they were still some distance away, Snowy felt the energy change and took off, spreading its broad wings over the top of the breakwater. I said farewell under my breath and decided to cut my swim short. I just didn't want to deal with those dogs.

DECEMBER 8, 2016

Today I ended my outdoor, mostly-in-Lake-O swimming streak: 591 consecutive days. I'd already made up my mind before I set out today: The forecasts are predicting real winter is arriving—in contrast to 2015, when the whole month of December had above-average temperatures. To be frank, I'm glad. I prefer real winter, especially the prospect of skating, by far my preferred way to commune with the water in winter. Wild skating is the only thing that gives me the same feeling as cold-water swimming. Freedom of movement, weightlessness, like flying. Communing with cold water in a different form.

I headed to Ward's Beach, knowing full well it would be windy and rough. It's never the water temp alone that gives me pause. It's the conditions, the before and after of the swim. Especially wind, cold, fierce wind. I just don't want to contend with them. Add to that the fact that the beach has become dog-walking central, and dogs make me nervous when I'm in the water, probably because the sight of someone in the water makes *them* nervous, antsy, and unpredictable, and for as long as I've been doing this cold-water swimming, I *hate* having people around when I do it. I just want to be alone, don't want to wonder whether they think I'm crazy, and can't stand the way they stop and point at me: "Can you believe it? There's someone swimming out there!" I don't know why I care. I shouldn't care. But I do.

I decided to check out the spot on First Street, on the harbor side, but it was just as rough and blustery. *For Chrissake*, I thought, *there's wind coming from all directions!* I headed along the gap to the beach, determined to go in, however briefly. Sure enough—dogs! Running and yapping along the shore, right in *my* spot near the Log Ness Monster. I headed to the western end of the beach to find a bit of shelter and to get away from the damn dogs. Just as I was about to go in, a couple of young guys came down the path. People! Thwarted at every turn.

The message of the day was clear: It's time to stop for the season. The streak ends today.

I waded in with my trusty pool thermometer: About 4 C (39 F), just what it should have been. I threw off my down jacket, strode out into the waves. At this end of the beach, the water is so shallow you have to go out about forty or fifty meters to get more than knee-deep. I didn't get that far. The wind was a bitch! I just flopped in up to my neck and let the waves slap me around a bit. Maybe stayed in for just over a minute, just as the two young men approached me.

"How's the water?" one asked.

"Cold," I replied. "Really cold."

Day 591, and that's a wrap!

CHAPTER 7

Profiles in Cold:
Ice milers and other extremists

One shouldn't be able to swim at the North
Pole in the first place.

—Lewis Pugh

LEWIS PUGH, known as "the Sir Edmund Hillary of swimming," is right. A person shouldn't be able to do what he
did in 2005, swim for nearly twenty minutes in water that
is -1.7 C (29 F). A human also shouldn't be able to swim
for more than two hours in 3.3 C (38 F) water, across the
Bering Strait from Alaska to Russia, as Lynne Cox did in
1987. People think cold-water swimmers must be crazy,
and that's more than a little bit true. But we ordinary mor-
tals aren't as crazy—or to put it more kindly, as toweringly
audacious—as these elite athletes.

This chapter is about cold-water swimming as an
extreme sport, and the conquerers who push the limits of

human ability and achieve the seemingly impossible. Pugh was the first person to swim across the icy waters of the North Pole. Concerned about the diminishing ice cover in the Arctic, his goal was to alert the world to the accelerating effects of climate change. Pugh's subsequent swims have had a similar environmental focus. In August 2014, he undertook a "Seven Seas" swim to draw attention to the health of the world's oceans. He swam 10 kilometers (about 6 miles) each in the Mediterranean, the Adriatic Sea, the Aegean Sea, the Black Sea, the Red Sea, the Persian Gulf, and the North Sea.

In 2018, Pugh outdid himself, swimming the entire length of the English Channel, the first person ever to do so. Issuing a call for one-third of the world's oceans to be protected by the year 2030, he spent 49 days at sea, swimming between 10 and 20 kilometers (6 to 12 miles) each day to cover the 528-kilometer (328-mile) distance.

Cox's achievements predate Pugh's by more than a decade. Her first major distance swim was across New Zealand's Cook Strait in 1975, when she was 18 years old. She has an arguably stronger claim to be the pioneer of what's been dubbed "Speedo diplomacy." It's a cliché that beauty-pageant contestants say their greatest wish is for world peace, but it's literally true for Cox, who helped bring about the end of the Cold War between the USA and the Soviet Union by swimming the Bering Strait in 1987. She wrote the following for the *New York Times*:

Few people believed anyone could survive for more than two hours in water that cold. The harder part was getting the Soviets to allow the swim at all. But my journey was the culmination of an 11-year effort to use sport to open the border between the United States and the Soviet Union. I wanted to make a difference.... Growing up during the Cold War, I was afraid that the tension and misunderstanding between the people of the United States and the Soviet Union would cause our mutual self-destruction. The smallest misstep between the superpowers could escalate into a world war.

Her accomplishment earned praise from both superpowers. At the signing of a major disarmament treaty at the White House, Soviet President Mikhail Gorbachev toasted Cox: "It took one brave American by the name of Lynne Cox just two hours to swim from one of our countries to the other. We saw on television how sincere and friendly the meeting was between our people and the Americans when she stepped onto the Soviet shore. She proved by her courage how close to each other our peoples live." Cox went on to numerous other accomplishments, most notably swimming more than a mile (1.6 kilometers) in the waters of Antarctica. Her book about the experience, *Swimming to Antarctica*, was published in 2004.

No surprise that both Pugh and Cox have done TED Talks and are in demand as inspirational speakers. They certainly inspired me; not to try and imitate them, but simply because I could point to them and say, "See? Swimming in cold water isn't crazy." I knew I didn't have the same ferocious inner drive that pushed Pugh and Cox beyond normal human limits. It's a calling. Even when they have nothing left to prove, elite athletes keep going, keep trying to top themselves. There is, of course, a perilous and often tragic side to this: Matthew Webb's doomed attempt to swim Niagara Falls in 1883 being the most famous example.

The extreme-sport mentality is seeping into the mainstream of cold-water swimming. After being coached by Lewis Pugh through a cold-water swim in a Welsh lake, British actor Robson Green called the experience "life changing. There was no swim I couldn't do after meeting Lewis because anything is possible if you *commit!*" That attitude concerns me, not only for the danger it can pose to an individual but for what it says about us as a society. Is it really true that "anything is possible" if you try hard enough? Is it all about "me" and "my triumphs?" Is modern life so easy that we have to search for challenges? Why would you want to risk harming your body to demonstrate that it's stronger than nature itself, which it demonstrably is not? Life is a gift, not a challenge. Even if you want to see it as a series of challenges, who needs to go looking for more? Isn't life tough enough already?

"THE INDIVIDUAL AGAINST HIMSELF"

Even in the dead of winter, people ask me, "How cold is the water?" I usually reply with something like, "Well, you can tell it's above zero, because it's still liquid." Mind you, fresh water freezes at 0 C (32 F) and salt water has a lower freezing temp, around -2 C (28.4 F). As I said earlier in this book, there has been the odd occasion when I've chipped through ice to get to water; but surely it goes without saying that "ice swimming" is a contradiction in terms. Well, someone had better tell the International Ice Swimming Association (IISA). Launched by South African extreme swimmer Ram Barkai in 2009, the IISA's focus is on activities in water 41 F (5 C) or colder. The chief raison d'être of the IISA is to promote and validate what it calls an ice mile: swimming a mile (about 1.6 kilometers) in water colder than 41 F (5 C), wearing only an ordinary swimsuit and bathing cap, known as English Channel rules. It's a sport that pits, as Barkai puts it, "the individual against himself," and draws on what he sees as a fundamental human drive: "Human nature is competitive and many focus on breaking records, else we would all be sitting in our caves, drawing charcoal on the walls." (Personally, I would argue that the work of cave artists was a far higher expression of human nature than any swimming record.)

The ice mile has been called the "Everest of cold-water swimming," and there's concern that, like Everest, it could attract participants who lack the necessary training and experience. From the IISA's earliest days, there have been questions about the fundamental safety of the ice-mile enterprise. Perhaps the fiercest critic has been Donal Buckley, who's devoted thousands of words to the subject on his LoneSwimmer blog. Buckley makes clear he doesn't want to ban the ice mile. In fact, he's completed one himself (more on that below). His concern is that the IISA guidelines don't convey the actual difficulty, in particular the very real life-threatening risks of attempting an ice mile. In 2014, IISA responded to Buckley and other critics by adding an ice kilometer event. (If you'll recall from your school days, a kilometer is a little more than half as long as a mile.) Everyone in the open-water swimming world knows that completing an ice kilometer carries a lower status than an ice mile—and the phrase "ice kilometer" is not as catchy. More recently, the IISA has taken the lead in pushing the International Olympic Committee to certify ice swimming as an Olympic sport, an effort that most in the open-water community view as a steep, uphill climb.

You'd think one organization would be enough in the ice-swimming world, but you'd be wrong. In fact, the International Winter Swimming Association (IWSA) predates the IISA by several years. Originating in Finland, IWSA events focus on three different conditions: cold water between 41 F and 48 F (5 C–9 C), with events up to 1,000 meters (0.6 mile) long; freezing water between 36 F and 41 F (2 C–5 C), with events up to 450 meters (0.28 mile) long, and "ice water" between 28 F and 36 F (-2 C–2 C), with events up to a maximum of 200 meters (0.1 mile) long. Clearly, the missions of the two organizations overlap, but they cooperate in some areas. For instance, they alternate annual sponsorship of the Winter Swimming World Championship. The main thing that differentiates them, not surprisingly, is the ice mile. The IWSA rejects the notion that any 1,000-meter swim in water under 5 C can be undertaken safely.

Despite his criticism of the IISA, Buckley decided that his credibility in the open-water swimming world demanded that he attempt one. He completed an ice mile in 2014, and the experience most definitely did not turn him into a fan: "The Ice Mile was awful, painful and horrible," he reported on his blog. "*Stupid and dangerous* is my preferred description of Ice Mile swimming." But his views haven't deterred many swimmers: Early in 2021, the number of certified ice milers climbed to more than four hundred worldwide. And with virtually all swimming moving outdoors during the pandemic, interest in the ice mile just keeps growing. There have no reports of deaths resulting from ice-mile attempts, but many swimmers have had post-swim difficulties, both immediate and long-term. Lynne Cox lost feeling in her hands for six months after her Bering Strait swim. After his extreme swims, Lewis Pugh experienced a similar loss of sensation in his hands.

The British scientist Heather Massey has emphasized there's a huge gap between the relative risk of taking a winter dip and attempting an ice mile. In the former, the swimmer monitors the changes in her body to avoid a cold-shock response. During an ice mile, however, the swimmer must actively ignore and push through those changes, even when they signal the onset of hypothermia. In an online panel on ice swimming in June 2021, sponsored by the World Open Water Swimming Association (WOWSA), Massey was joined by Mike Tipton, Ram Barkai and Dr. Otto Thaning. Thaning, a thoracic surgeon, trained under Dr. Christiaan Barnard, who carried out the first heart transplant in 1967. Like Tipton and Massey, Thaning is also a cold-water swimmer who, in 2014, aged sixty-four, became the oldest person to cross the English Channel. So all the panelists had first-hand involvement in cold-water activities, yet they all agreed, to varying degrees, on the very real risks. Thaning raised the possibility that extreme cold-water immersion might cause an abnormal heart rhythm, triggering pulmonary edema and even death. Other panelists weighed in on the spectre of permanent nerve damage to the extremities, especially hands and fingers. Barkai confided he had once advised a concert pianist to "stay away from ice swimming" for that very reason.

I'm no stranger to ice. On occasion I've broken through it for a swim. One time, I swam around floating sheets of ice in Lake Louise, a gorgeous glacier-fed lake in the Canadian Rockies, where a group of tourists applauded as I emerged from the water. I briefly entertained the idea of shooting for an ice mile myself. I've already made clear that I'm a slow swimmer, and my long-distance ambitions never came to fruition; but this sounded like something I could do. Swimming a mile is no biggie for me—I've done it. And the bragging rights would far outweigh my 365-day swim. Maybe, like Donal Buckley, I thought people expected me to try it.

I delved into online accounts of the experiences of ice-mile swimmers, and learned that they frequently emerge from the water disoriented, unable to walk, with no control of their limbs, completely dependent on their support team to get dressed and rewarmed. Some describe "blanking out" during the final stage of the swim, losing all memory of leaving the water and rewarming. Hallucinations are also common toward the end of the swim. One of the most frightening is what Buckley calls "black rain," spots in front of his eyes that increased in size, speed and seeing distance, accompanied by other visual disturbances and loss of peripheral vision. Another prominent ice swimmer accidentally left his goggles behind on one of his first ice swims and suffered temporary blindness. Black rain? Frozen eyeballs? Um, no. I'll take care of the one good eye I have, thanks very much.

I felt a growing sense of relief as I found more and more reasons to discard the prospect of an ice swim and the intense training it would involve. (You already know how I feel about *training*.) It took four letters to snap me out it once and for all: NFCI, which stands for "non-freezing cold injury." If that sounds like an awfully vague diagnosis, that's because so little is known about what it actually is. A condition mostly confined to military settings (at least until ice swimmers came along), NFCI is distinct from frostbite. It affects the extremities of the body, including the hands or feet, due to exposure to wet conditions that are above freezing. Blood flow is blocked to the affected parts of the body, causing the fingers or toes to go white and numb. It can lead to permanent nerve damage and other debilitating conditions, such as Raynaud's Syndrome. Mike Tipton calls NFCI the "hidden threat" for cold-water swimmers because it only appears after, sometimes *long* after, the actual swim. The presence of the word "permanent" strikes terror in my soul. I write with my hands. I play music with my hands. Why would I engage in an activity that could jeopardize my ability to do those things?

The comparison with Everest is apt. More than three hundred people have died attempting to climb the mountain, and in recent decades that number has soared, with many climbers who were inexperienced and underprepared. Like Everest, the ice mile is fraught with danger, an extreme sport that properly belongs in the domain of elite athletes. Still, I'm of two minds. Cold-water swimmers are an awfully independent-minded bunch. I've certainly never wanted anyone to tell me what I could or couldn't do in the water. One of the first Canadian women to complete an ice mile says she found the whole experience by turns "exciting, hormonal, frustrating, dangerous, intoxicating, and empowering." Katharine Borczak is one of a trio of women who set out to, in her words, "put Canadian women on the map" of ice-mile swimming in 2018. "It was the best thing I did for myself as a woman that year. I learned I was resilient in the harshest environments." Like many ice milers, Borczak had a difficult recovery, and experienced numbness in her extremities for months after the swim; but she has no regrets: "I would rather swim thirty-nine minutes in 4 C temp than run 42 kilometers in blistering heat." Borczak has since become a key mentor in the cold-water community, encouraging and supporting other swimmers through her Facebook group Canadian Cold Water Swimming.

THE ICEMAN

I'd been well into my cold-water addiction for several years when a neighbor asked me whether I was a follower of Wim Hof.

I shook my head. "What's that?"

It turned out that he was talking about a person.

"Wim Hof. You've got to check him out. He's the Iceman!"

I assured him I would. My first thought was to wonder about that catchy, hashtag-worthy name, which I assumed was made up. But googling those six letters brought up a veritable flood of links to websites, magazine articles, videos, and photos of a bearded Dutchman in a variety of cold environments—glaciers, mounds of snow, tubs of ice cubes—wearing nothing but a pair of shorts. Looking at the photos, even I was like, "Why would anyone want to do that?" Clearly, among cold aficionados, this Wim Hof fellow was in a class by himself.

Hof has set more cold-exposure records than anyone can keep track of, including several world records for the longest time in direct, full-body contact with ice. He achieves this by sitting in tubs full of ice cubes, and his personal best time hovers in the neighborhood of two hours. His Instagram handle is *@iceman_hof*, and some of his feats have a gimmicky quality: running a half marathon barefoot on ice and snow; climbing Everest and Kilimanjaro wearing nothing but shorts and shoes. But Hof is dead serious about showcasing his near-superhuman abilities. He claims he can consciously control his core body temperature, and has subjected himself to extensive testing to prove it. Medical experts don't claim to understand how he does it, but they say something unusual is going on in Hof's body.

At least in part, that's because his approach springs from a very different source than ice swimmers and other extreme athletes. It's more of a spiritual discipline than a challenge and needs to be viewed in the context of Hof's compelling personal story. His first wife Olaya's suicide in 1995 started him on a quest to deal with his own grief, and ultimately led to a system and book called *The Wim Hof Method* (WHM). It involves three "pillars:" cold exposure; meditation; and breathing techniques with similarities to Tummo, an "inner fire" breathing practice, rooted in Tibetan Buddhism. The WHM has thousands of followers worldwide who practice the three pillars in a variety of ways. People who live in warmer climes and can't get to a body of cold water use cold showers. Hof's website and Facebook page feature photos of adherents demonstrating their cold-exposure techniques. Sitting in chest freezers full of ice cubes is popular.

The other two pillars aren't as photo-friendly, of course, and some medical experts are concerned about the safety of the breathing practices. A more general criticism of the WHM—true of many other wellness regimens, as well—is that its benefits are oversold. Is it all about money? Hard to say. You can pay for online courses and even weekend retreats led by the man himself, but it's no more questionable than paying for personal trainers and meditation retreats. And a lot of the basic WHM information is freely available. If the Facebook group page is any indication, the followers of Wim Hof are a mixed bag of spiritual seekers, macho show-offs, and deeply distressed people looking for miracle cures. Clearly, many find what they're looking for in the WHM.

As I've become more connected to the cold-water universe, I've noticed a certain kind of social-media behavior common among cold-immersion enthusiasts. Swimmers post before and after selfies, with captions listing the distance they swam, the amount of time spent in the water and, most importantly, the water temperature, often accompanied by a snapshot of a digital thermometer. It's a harmless bit of bragging. Cold-water swimmers can all relate to the pride of doing something the rest of the population finds so difficult. Cold-water newbies are the most enthusiastic posters, but it's a habit that's mostly foreign to early adopters—like the daily dippers in the Ladies and Men's Ponds of London, who've been plunging into cold water was long before the days of social media. It's telling that there isn't much interest in the WHM among elite swimmers. In fact, many cold-water veterans find it annoying that Wim Hof has become the public face of cold exposure as a health regimen.

Nowadays, things readily tip over into competitiveness:

cold-water swimming as a test of endurance. You must always be going colder, swimming farther, staying in longer, attempting to achieve something no one else has done—which, these days, has become well-nigh impossible. At its extreme, it's a fetishization of the idea that the body has no limits, that "there's nothing you can't do if you set your mind to it." But this is a mantra for extreme athletes, not ordinary people. More than once, it's made me feel inadequate, until I remind myself that it isn't a performance, that I go into cold water for my own pleasure and well-being. This farther-colder-longer attitude is especially common among male swimmers. So, I was pleased to hear a very different message—that the body *does* have its limits!—from a cold-water champion, and a female swimmer to boot.

"IT'S NOT ABOUT THE SWIM"

The first time that I saw Nuala Moore finish an Ice Kilometer in a falling snow after she had completed 40 laps in the 25m pool carved out of a frozen lake in Burghausen, Germany, I knew she was one of the world's most well-adapted cold water swimmers.... She was just standing there after finishing her swim in 2°C water. She wasn't shivering, she was smiling. She wasn't cold, she was cheerful. She didn't bother to even jump in the hot tub, she just continued to cheer for her Irish teammates and swimmers from all over the world.

As is clear from this admiring comment from fellow elite swimmer Steve Munatones, the woman who hails from Ireland's rugged Dingle Peninsula is no slouch. For more than a decade, Nuala Moore has swum in water temperatures as low as 0 C (32 F). Her journey to the ice began in 2012, when she competed in Siberia in -33 C (27 F) air temperature. In 2013, she completed a one-kilometer ice swim in Murmansk, Russia, and has since set ice-swimming distance records in Ireland and around the world. More recently, Moore's focus has shifted more toward other swimmers rather than trying to outdo her own records. She's become an evangelist for safety in cold-water swimming and her mantra, "It's not about the swim," reflects her conviction that the human being in the water is far more important than the mechanics of swimming: "This is a danger zone and we have to step up…. It's not a matter of 'if' the cold will take us, it's a matter of 'when' the cold completely stops us," she wrote on the WOWSA blog page in late 2020. "The sea/lakes are not confined swimming pools, you don't get to stand up when you have a problem. It's understanding the rules will keep you safe."

In 2016, Moore wrote a manual, *An Insight into the World of Ice Swimming*, incorporating research and discussion with Russian medical teams with which she'd collaborated, and went on to become a practitioner of ocean extreme medicine, with a focus on cold-water injuries. This work took on great urgency during the Pandemic as pool closures and the resulting boom in open-water swimming spiked the need for rescues. Moore says many of them could have been avoided with education. "Regardless of your swim level, regardless of whether you spend ten minutes or two hours in the water, if we swim in cold water, there is a need for us all to manage our outcomes. We cannot enter the water without a plan to be safe. Cold water has limits and so do we." One of Moore's pet phrases about cold-water swimming is, "When in doubt, get out."

Moore's work in water safety is relevant not just for extreme swimmers. More people are immersing in cold water for relief from various conditions, physical and mental. Many find it reduces their suffering, and there's growing evidence that cold-water immersion can relieve anxiety and depression. The practice has a long history: According to Roger Deakins, depression was one of the main conditions that people sought treatment for during the nineteenth-century spa boom. Nowadays, sufferers from emotional distress are finding mutual support through cold-water activities and they're sharing their experiences through Facebook groups such as Mental Health Swims and Swimming4Sanity. It turns out that social media isn't just for boasting about cold-water exploits.

Cold-water swimming has long been, and will likely continue to be, something of an outlaw pastime. A group I follow on Facebook recently had a spirited discussion on the merits of various tools for cutting into an icy pond. (The debate narrowed down to a chainsaw vs. something called a Scandinavian ice saw.) There's even growing interest in the sport of diving under ice, a prospect that makes even my blood run cold. And, as hard as it might have been to imagine, cold-water swimming has emerged as an opportunity for corporate branding. A new company called ICEWIM is marketing "the first swimwear for cold-water swimmers" made from what it calls an eco-friendly substitute for neoprene. Cold water is even finding a place in pop culture: Comedian Kevin Hart has a sports talk show where he interviews guests while they both sit in tubs of ice water. The show's title is "Cold as Balls."

As I've searched for my place in the cold-water universe, I've come to realize that it's not about competition or testing physical limits or trying to achieve nirvana. I'm in the Roger Deakins' camp: I'm more a bather than a swimmer, more interested in experiencing aquatic life than in overcoming it. I'm no guru, and I don't want to be anyone's acolyte. It's really quite simple: I go in cold water because of the way it makes me feel. In a very real sense, my life revolves around getting into the water, no matter how far I am from home, as the next chapter makes clear.

CHAPTER 8

Where's the Water?
My watery travels

IN THE EARLY 2000s, I spent a month taking part in a theater workshop at the University of Lethbridge, in Alberta. It was my first time on the Canadian prairies. Though Alberta doesn't have as much of the grassy flatlands and endless skies of Manitoba or Saskatchewan, it was a different terrain than I was used to. The first few days, I got to know my way around campus but kept having an odd feeling, as though I was looking for something, and couldn't put my finger on what it was. One day I was biking from the University to the city center along Whoop-Up Drive (named after a nineteenth-century whisky trading post) and found myself on a bridge. There it was, below me: water! The Old Man River (yes, really). I wasn't nearly as fanatical about outdoor swimming as I am now, and I had no thought of actually going into the river but at least knew where it was.

It's a lifelong preoccupation. Wherever I go, I wonder: Where's the water? Something in me is always searching for water; it's a fundamental part of my mental geography. Nowadays, when I'm in a new place, I feel it with more urgency than ever: Where's the water? There's usually water somewhere in the vicinity—a lake, a river, a pond—and I need to know where it is in order to orient myself. I've never wanted to go to the desert or any bone-dry environment. The thought is distressing.

As I've grown older, the chance for a near-daily immersion in water has become more and more important. Whenever I travel I'm always thinking: Where can I swim today? It wasn't a problem when our daughters were growing up. Our family holidays always involved access to water: visiting family on the Nova Scotia coast; canoe tripping in pristine northern lakes. On car trips I'd look for any sign of water on road maps, so we could stop for a quick dip. Over time, proximity to water became the focus of any traveling I did, which is how I found myself on a "swimming holiday" in Croatia, in the summer of 2014.

BIG RIVER MAN AND SON

My spouse Alec and I planned a trip to Italy that summer. Alec, who's fluent in Italian, had been there several times on work-related trips. The one time I'd accompanied him a couple of years earlier I found that, while it was wonderful having an interpreter, I spent a lot of time on the sidelines of animated conversations he was having with his colleagues. This time, we'd be spending most of the time away from the coast, so the swimming prospects weren't great. I realized I needed to do something on my own. But what?

Then I saw *Big River Man*, a hilarious, disturbing, awe-inspiring film about long-distance swimmer Martin Strel that chronicles his 2007 swim of the Amazon. I was amazed to learn that, before his death, Charles Sprawson was working on a biography of Strel. It's hard to imagine a greater contrast than that between the refined, introverted Sprawson and the Falstaffian, beer-bellied Strel; but open-water swimming attracts individualists, and Strel is nothing if not a larger-than-life personality. I learned about Strel Swimming, a company founded by Martin and his son Borut, that organizes swimming holidays. The whole notion was new to me, but clearly the Strel name gave them a head start in what was then a fledgling industry. The family hails from Slovenia (which I then knew mainly as the home of Melania Trump), but Borut conducted summer trips from a base in neighboring Croatia, just across the Adriatic from the Veneto area of Italy. The website hinted that, on occasion, participants might get to meet the Big River Man himself. I scrolled through and found a five-day "Island-Hopping" trip that fit my schedule and budget.

Croatia has a long, gorgeous coastline, with stunningly clear water and thousands of islands. For this trip, our home base was Krapanj, an island with a history of sponge diving, about an hour's drive and short boat ride from the city of Split. We were booked at a nice hotel—almost too nice, I thought. Weren't we here to do fierce exercise, to challenge ourselves? After checking in, I took a walk down the long quay lined with outdoor cafés and bistros, and noticed that at almost every table people were drinking an orange concoction in large round goblets. Over the course of the week, I learned the drink was an Aperol spritz, a mixture of prosecco and a bittersweet, bright-orange aperitif that was the locals' near-universal choice for cocktail hour. (In the spirit of "when in Rome"—or in this case, Croatia—the Aperol spritz became a lasting favorite of my own.)

The daily pattern was set the next morning: A dozen of us gathered on the quay, boarded a boat and headed out to the spot Borut had picked for our morning swim. After lunch on the boat, we took off again for an afternoon swimming spot, then headed back to the hotel on Krapanj. The Strel website said we'd be swimming an average of 4 kilometers (2.5 miles) a day. Having done several distance swims, I knew that wouldn't be a problem. I was glad there was no mention of speed. Sometimes we swam along a shoreline, other times we did a crossing between two islands. I never felt alone or unsafe in the water. Two inflatable Zodiacs escorted the swimmers, and the main boat was never out of sight. Plus we were always clearly visible with our hot-pink and electric-yellow swim caps. Once we had to bail on what was supposed to be a 3-kilometer (1.8-mile) swim because Borut said the wind and waves made it too hard to control the big boat for pick-ups.

After the first morning, Borut divided us into two groups—the really good swimmers, who always started swimming first, and the ordinary swimmers (guess which group I was in?) who were ferried ahead of the first group before jumping in—the idea being that we'd all finish at roughly the same time. This never happened. The fast swimmers always overtook us, and it became an incentive for me not to keep them waiting too long. The group was almost all female, mostly Brits, a handful of other Europeans, and a few Aussies, one of whom had swum the English Channel. The whole scene was reminiscent of high school: The fast swimmers were the "popular" kids, the pretty-good swimmers were in the middling ranks, and the slowbies were the nerds. I wasn't always dead last, though sometimes that was because the women would stop swimming and chat while I kept on going. I was the oldest in the group, and at first they didn't quite know what to make of me, this slow-swimming Canadian. But I held my own, and never bailed on a swim. In the end, this won me a measure of respect, even from the Channel swimmer herself.

Through the week Borut had been unfailingly positive ("Great swim!" or "You're doing very well!") It was the kind of vacuous praise I normally can't stand, but out there on the water, I appreciated it. Maybe I was a decent swimmer, after all. Slow but steady, right? On the last day, we were each filmed underwater as we swam. The footage would be shown later that night at a closing, stroke-assessment session. I wasn't sure I liked the sound of that and approached the final night with trepidation. I sat waiting my turn, hoping that Borut would say something like, "Kathleen, you're slow, but you have very nice form." But no. Turns out I didn't have nice form at all: my fingers were splayed; my legs were a literal drag; my stroke was "inefficient." Borut's critiques were all delivered in a positive spirit, with the intent to help us correct mistakes and improve our technique. But I wasn't really sure how hard I wanted to *work* at my swimming.

Fortunately, "swimming holiday" turned out to be an accurate description, because we did some interesting tourist-y things too. One day we visited the ruins of a sixth-century Byzantine fortress, built during the reign of Emperor Justinian. Another time, we stopped at an island where there had been a youth camp and resort during the Soviet era. Since abandoned, the island was now home to a single hermit and his dog. It was an eerie place, full of empty buildings and twisting paths paved in concrete. At the edge of the water were the remains of what looked like an amphitheatre, with circular stone walls and rows of steps. Nearby, was an old wash pavilion with a row of crumbling sinks, piles of old tubing, even a few shoes. One night, the group went into Šibenik, a beautiful medieval town, for dinner at a konoba, a kind of tavern with food. It was right at the edge of the town square, where there were scads of kids running around, riding bikes, playing till well after dark—the kind of freewheeling childhood that North Americans wax nostalgic for. As we were leaving, the kids were sitting on rows of stone steps watching a movie projected on a good, old-fashioned portable screen.

I never did get to meet the Big River Man. And as much as I enjoyed seeing that part of the world and being in the water every day, I knew I wouldn't be back anytime soon. I realized anew what a freshwater girl I am, and how important the temperature factor is to me. As lovely as the Adriatic is, the water is just too damn warm.

THE OUTLAW SWIMMERS OF EUROPE

There's one place I've visited where there's absolutely no need to ask, "Where's the water?" In Venice, you can't avoid it. When we visited there in the early twenty-teens, I found it strangely unsettling to be constantly surrounded by water—which might sound odd, coming from someone who professes to love it so much. But that was precisely the source of my distress. I said earlier that I'm one of those people who can't see a body of water without wanting to jump in. *Wanting* isn't the same as *doing*, of course. As much as I enjoyed the glories of the historic city, I found I really had to work to tamp down that impulse while in Venice. We were only there a few days, and I did manage to have one decent swim at the beach on the Venice Lido. I knew I'd be stopped if I even tried to swim in the city, but I was seized by a thought: What about a quick dip in one of the side canals? There was a stairway down to one of them in the apartment we'd rented. It was too narrow for boat traffic or even a sidewalk, and largely hidden from sight. On our last day, I put on a swimsuit, descended the stairs and lowered myself into the water. (Don't worry, I didn't put my head under.) In all the adventure lasted no more than a minute. I barely got wet and, to be honest, I only dipped in the canal it so I could *say* I did it.

Thus began my mischievous career as an Outlaw swimmer in Europe.

Unlike Venice, my next foray into forbidden waters had a purpose—to cool off in the stifling heat of summer in Rome. I'd heard there was a pool near the Colosseum that was open (for a hefty price) to the public, but for some reason it was closed while we were there. I remember standing in the crowd near the Trevi Fountain in muggy 34 C (93 F) heat, longing to take a *La Dolce Vita*-style plunge. Later, as evening approached, Alec and I were walking along the Tiber and I spied a stone stairway leading to a concrete platform on the riverbank. It looked to be a loading zone for tour boats but it was empty. When we walked down, I saw the water level was high enough for an easy scramble back onto the platform. It was quite dark, and we were well below street level. I stripped to my underwear and quietly slipped in. No one noticed. The night was so warm that my clothes were mostly dry by the time we got back to our apartment in Trastevere.

"NO SWIMMING" IN BELGIUM

Belgium is where I really earned my outlaw-swimmer badge. Alec and I spent a few days in Bruges—and yes, there's a movie with that very title. If you've seen it or been there yourself, you know that Bruges is a small city full of gorgeous medieval buildings, cobblestone streets and, most importantly for the purposes of this book, canals! Once directly connected with the sea, gradual silting since the eleventh century has caused Bruges to lose direct access to open water. The town is sometimes referred to as the Venice of the North, and though the canals aren't as ubiquitous as in Venice, I found them much more inviting. I scoped for possible points of entry as we walked along one, near where we were staying, and was pleased to see sturdy metal ladders placed about 50 meters (164 feet) apart all along the quay. I made my way down and proceeded to have a delightful, honest-to-goodness swim. A few people watched with curiosity, but with no outrage that I could discern. It was only as I climbed back up the ladder that I saw the bright red, text-free sign. We were in the

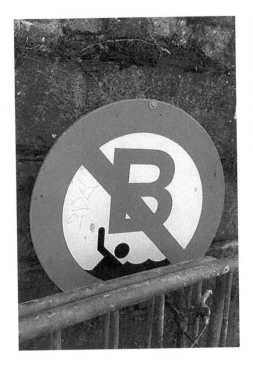

"'No Swimming' (which I disobeyed). Bruges, Belgium (2017)."
Photo by Kathleen McDonnell.

Francophone part of Belgium, so I knew exactly what the line through big B stood for: *pas de baignade*, or "stay out of the water!" There had been no such signage on the Tiber or in Venice, probably because it was considered unnecessary. I mean, who in their right mind would think of swimming in such places?

Ah, Paris. People go there for the cafés, the baguettes, the art galleries and museums, and to fall in love...but to swim? Yes, and by now you shouldn't be the least bit surprised.

Over a period of a dozen years, I made a number of trips to France to research an earlier book, *Swim Home: Searching for the Wild Girl of Champagne*. (Yes, I've written two books with titles that reference swimming.) It's a historical detective story recounting my somewhat-obsessive search for the truth about a famous feral child, Marie-Angélique LeBlanc, who was found in the Champagne district nearly three hundred years ago. One of the things that drew me to her story was the fact that she loved to swim, not an approved activity for ladies in eighteenth-century France. Early accounts from the estate where she lived for a time tell of the servants' efforts to keep her from diving into the moat. That estate, complete with moat, is now a winery, and in the book I recount how the current proprietors tried to discourage me from plunging in as well. "*C'est trop froid!*" one insisted. My French wasn't adequate to explain my cold-water swimming practices, so I just assured them they shouldn't worry: "*Je suis Canadienne!*"

I managed to spend a few days in Paris during those research trips. I'd heard about something called *Paris Plages*, where the city had created a huge public swimming area accessible from a floating platform in the Seine. It was in the portion of the river known as *Le Bassin de la Villette*, and I was itching to swim there. Alas, it was open only during the summer, and the season had ended by the time I arrived in 2017. Apparently, a few people continued to swim there after the pool area was officially closed, and city authorities mostly turned a blind eye. I was too timid to venture into an illegal situation in a foreign country and, reluctantly, took a pass.

Later, I stumbled across an even more intriguing fact: People swam in the Catacombs, the complex network of tunnels underneath the city, despite being strictly forbidden by Paris authorities. To my mind, these adventurers were the ultimate outlaw swimmers, and I searched to find a way to connect with them for my next trip. Then I got the real scoop on the Catacombs from a friend. Journalist Marco Oved of the *Toronto Star* had previously freelanced in Paris, and he produced a radio documentary about the cave adventurers, known as cataphiles. According to Marco, swimming in the Paris Catacombs was a misnomer. I would have had to crawl through dark, claustrophobic tunnels on my hands and knees just to get to waist-deep water, which didn't sound like fun at all. Another pass.

In 2018, I was preparing to make what likely would be the last research trip for my *Wild Girl of Champagne* book. This time I was determined to swim in the Seine. I learned about a group called *Laboratoire des baignades urbaines expérimentales* (Laboratory of Experimental Urban Swimming) that, despite its official-sounding name, was a renegade movement to reclaim Paris waterways for year-round swimming. In the words of one of the founders, Alex Voyer, "French culture has taught us to fight with authority, and that's why we like to enjoy these beautiful waterways that are available to us." They started hearing from more and more people who wanted to join, so Voyer set up a Facebook group called Paris Wild Swimming. Whatever you might think of it as a social media site, one of the glories of Facebook is how it connects people with common interests. In recent years, open-water swimming has spawned a worldwide community. In almost any corner of the world, it's easy to connect with local swimmers. They can give you the lowdown on where and when the next group swim is happening. It's a bit like speed-dating for swimmers.

That was how I ended up beside the *Canal de l'Ourcq*, on the northeastern edge of the city. Part of a network of canals built in the ninetheeth century, the out-of-the-way location appeals to its regular swimmers, who call themselves *Les Ourcq Polaires*, to avoid the attention of Paris' gendarmerie. After carefully studying Google Maps and the daunting maze of the Paris Métro, I arrived at the appointed spot on the quay to meet two men and a woman, who welcomed me warmly as their new outlaw swimming friend. Everyone introduced themselves, but I promptly forgot their names except for Eddy, the one who'd replied to my Facebook post. We'd all donned swimsuits under our clothes, and began to strip down. I was a bit concerned as I scanned the wall along the canal, noting the lack of a good entry and exit point. But the woman pulled a rolled-up object out of her knapsack and proceeded to tie one end of it to an iron cleat on the quay. A portable rope ladder! I resolved then and there to buy one when I got back to Canada. Eddy was first in and said he wanted to make sure I could manage the cold water. I asked what the temperature was, and he replied about 13 C (55 F). "*Pas de problème!*" I laughed, as I headed down the rope ladder. The four of us spent a good twenty minutes swimming up and down the canal. We attracted the bemused attention of strollers on the quay but nothing to suggest we were doing anything particularly unusual. Afterwards, I noticed my companions were expert at changing from their swimsuits into dry clothes without revealing much flesh, a skill honed by open-water swimmers the world over! After a swim, some groups go out together for a drink, but it was early in the day and these folks had stuff to do, which was just as well since the weakness of my conversational French would have been laid bare within moments. I thanked them profusely, as we all went our separate ways. Later in the day, I came across a chic below-ground cocktail bar near my apartment, and toasted myself. At long last, I'd had an outdoor swim in Paris, just not in the main arm of the Seine, which would have to wait for another trip.

ICELAND: WHERE ARE ALL THE SWIMMERS?

In 2017, Alec and I decided to take advantage of a stopover deal from Icelandair on our way to Ireland. For the same cost as a round-trip fare, we could stop and spend several days in Iceland at one end of the trip. I was certain this three-day stopover was going to be the highlight of my swimming adventures to date. What could be more appealing for a cold-water swimmer than a country whose name was Iceland? Arriving in Reykjavík, I was struck by the constant presence of blue sea wherever I looked. As in Venice, there was water, water, everywhere, but no obvious indication of where to swim. Our apartment was close to a wharf, so on our first day we walked past the fishing boats and sightseeing vessels down to the shoreline, which was blocked by a wall of huge boulders. At a few spots, I could see small beaches where one could walk into the water. But there was no way to get to them other than by scrambling over the rock wall. Scrambling over rocks was never a strong point for someone as balance-challenged as I am, and it didn't look like the locals made a habit of it either.

I'd read about Nauthólsvík, a geothermal beach where one has the choice of sitting in a hot tub, swimming in a thermally heated natural pool, or taking a plunge in the cold seawater—or all of the above, in succession. That sounded great to me, but Nauthólsvík was some distance from where we were staying. Worse, I learned that the beach had switched to winter hours, in the middle of August, and was open only for a couple of hours in the afternoon. We were well into our second day of the stopover by then and wouldn't be able to get there before closing time. I decided to check out one of the year-round pools for which Reykjavík is famous. Vesturbæjarlaug (don't ask me how to pronounce it) turned out to be, well, just a pool, barely long enough at 30 meters (98 feet) for a decent lane swim. It had been more than a year since I'd swum in a pool, and the experience was as disappointing as ever: too warm (about 26 C or 79 F) with the monotonous turns at each end, driving home the reality that you're *not going anywhere.*

Worst of all, the chlorine. Pools in Iceland are supposedly "lightly" chlorinated, hence the strictly observed pre-swim ritual of a naked soap-all-over shower. But as far as I could tell, Vesturbæjarlaug had the same amount of chlorine as a typical North American pool. In fact, with a family play pool and a large round hot tub, it wasn't much different from the average chain-hotel pool. Any swim, even in a chlorine-blue rectangle, was better than no swim, but I was disillusioned. Where were the hardy Icelandic water lovers I'd heard so much about?

The next day, we resolved to get out of the city and rented a car to drive what the tourist board calls the Golden Circle. Our main destination was Þingvellir National Park (apparently the odd-looking first letter is pronounced like "th"), which contains a huge freshwater lake. As we drove along its shore, I was practically drooling at the prospect of a cool plunge in fresh water. But once again, the water was there and the trick was getting to it. Large plains of lichen-covered rock lay between the shoreline and the road, and no turn-offs or points of entry presented themselves. Once we entered the park and got out to walk the paths, the lake was even farther away. Small pools and a stream emptied into a river, which flowed into the lake in the distance. It gradually dawned on me that if I was going to get my full-body water fix, it would have to be in the river. We found a spot where a small sandy area offered access to the water. There were no signs forbidding swimming, and I'd learned that Icelanders are not at all shy about posting rules and restrictions of various sorts, but there was no one in the water. Clearly, it just wasn't done, and I probably risked a stern reprimand if I did it. Even more intimidating was the river's current, which was moving quite swiftly—not strong enough to sweep me away, but I didn't want to do something that might create an incident. Still, the sun was warm and I was hot from hiking, so I stripped down to my swimsuit. A quick dip would do the trick.

The river was, as I expected, quite shallow and had a soft, muddy bottom. If I'd dared to venture out into the middle I could've reached deeper water, but decided it was unwise, given the current. So I slid my body under the surface of the water just long enough to enjoy the cold, clean bite of it, then crawled back onto the shore. I was swimming in mud, and not for the first time. (Once, on a hot day in the south of France, I found a small lake on the map and asked Alec to pull off the road so I could take a quick dip. The "lake" was maybe 16 inches, or 40 centimeters, deep and yes, it was mud. All mud, and not even cool and refreshing like the one in Þingvellir.)

The rest of our Golden Circle jaunt included stops at Gulfoss, an astoundingly powerful waterfall, and Geysir, a site of hot springs, one of which spewed a 30-foot (9-meter) tower of boiling water every few minutes. Wonderful water experiences, but neither (obviously) beckoned for a plunge.

The next day was spent in Reykyavík and I made a second any-port-in-a-storm visit to the pool at Vesturbæjarlaug. Since we were booked to fly home the next day, it didn't look like I was going to get my cold-water fix in Iceland after all. But when I woke up the next morning, the sun was shining and I was seized with a thought that, amazingly, hadn't occurred to me before. Our flight didn't leave until 5 p.m. We had time to kill! The fabled Nauthólsvík Geothermal Beach would be open from 11 a.m. to 1 p.m. We could pack up, grab a taxi with our luggage in tow, and still have plenty of time to catch the bus to the airport.

The driver smiled when I told him we wanted to go to the thermal beach with the name beginning with "N." We drove past the municipal airport toward the sea, and pulled up to a lot surrounded by modern buildings.

"It's over there," the driver said, pointing to a concrete walkway. I couldn't see any evidence of a beach, just more piles of rocks and boulders. Then I saw him—a thickset, middle-aged man wearing a skimpy bikini brief, dripping wet, emerging at the top of a stone stairway. We got out and looked over the concrete wall. There were dozens of people in the water—all shapes, ages, sizes, some standing in waist-high water, some lounging in a long rectangular hot tub, chatting. But out beyond the roped-off area, the open ocean loomed, and there they were. Dozens of people! Some swimming, some bobbing leisurely, but all fully immersed. I could see on their faces the buzzing grins that only comes with one thing: Finally, I had found my people, the cold-water lovers of Iceland.

We couldn't risk missing our flight, but I *had* to get into that water, even if only for a few minutes. I don't know what the water temp was, I'd estimate about 8 C (46 F). (I've become something of a human thermometer, trying to guess then measure.) There was no time to join the folks soaking leisurely in the hot tub, but that didn't matter. Nauthólsvík was my glorious reward, at the end of a long search.

IRELAND BY WATER

As connected as I felt to the cold-water swimmers of Iceland, my true water-loving kindred are in a country whose name involves the switch of only one letter. The Irish don't just love the water, they can't stay *out* of the water. I got my first inkling that being Irish explained my cold-water obsession one day on Ward's Beach. An Irishman, who was visiting a neighbor, was just entering the water as I came out. We'd exchanged nods a couple of times before, but now I could see he was a swimming comrade. As I passed him on the shore I mentioned that the lake was a bit colder than on the previous day. He stopped me.

"Oh, no. We never use the word 'cold.'"

His lilting accent sounded mischievous, but he was completely serious.

"We just say 'it's gone down a degree or two.'"

I laughed. "Yeah, that's a good way to put it."

What he meant, of course, was something I came to learn in the course of my swimming exploits: that the experience of water temperature is, more than anything, all in the mind. Of course it's abundantly physical too— human flesh in contact with liquid whose temperature can be measured accurately with a thermometer. But how the water *feels* on the skin is subjective and largely determined by one's expectations. Typically, people run into the water expecting to feel cold. They shriek and hug their shoulders to brace themselves, but they're going about it the wrong way. Tensing up ensures the water will feel cold. My new Irish acquaintance was advocating a simple strategy: Don't *think* cold. Avoid the very word cold. Don't let it enter your head. I knew this instinctively, but I didn't know other people knew it, certainly not an entire nation (as I'm sure he meant by "we"). I was awakening to the fact that the Irish were not just my blood kin, but my swimming kin as well.

Perhaps the most compelling evidence of their propensity for water is the willingness of the Irish to jump into their most fabled river and swim a mile and a half (2.4 kilometers). The Liffey Swim is an annual race in Dublin's main river, dating back more than a century. Yes, it's a race, with timekeepers and medal winners, but it's also a communal gathering of water lovers, most of whom are psychrolutes. This is a no-wetsuit event in temperatures averaging 14 C (57 F). When I participated in 2016, it felt as though I was submerging myself in the baptismal waters of my ancestors. I was one of more than four hundred swimmers wearing the race's official hot-pink swimcap, which I still have. We were divided into men's and women's heats, and took turns entering the water from floating pontoons in the river. Although I didn't know any of the women in my heat, their camaraderie was infectious. As each group took the plunge, they joined in singing what's become the unofficial anthem of Dublin:

In Dublin's fair city, where the girls are so pretty
'Twas there that I met my sweet Molly Malone
She drove her wheelbarrow through the streets broad
and narrow
Crying "cockles and mussels, alive, alive, oh."

To me, it all felt a bit chaotic, though it didn't seem so to most of the swimmers who were regulars, familiar with the drill. Between the current and the other swimmers, I found the water choppy and never quite found a rhythm. The route was punctuated by a number of bridges over the river, and it was exhilarating to swim under each one with the cheering crowds overhead. Every so often, a surge of pink caps would surround me, swimmers in the later heats, catching up to the slow early starters like yours truly. Sooner than I expected, I spied the big, blue inflatable arch that marked the finish line. I found it a fairly easy swim, despite the choppiness, probably due to the strong current and the tidal flow. Some swimmers had clustered around the base of the stone stairway, waiting their turn to emerge from the water. As I started my ascent, I was pleased to see there were still a few pink caps in the water behind me. I'd managed to avoid finishing dead last! At the top of the stairway, a couple of guys greeted and congratulated each and every swimmer. One took my hand and the other asked how I was doing. "I'm good," I replied. With a cluster of other swimmers, I proceeded through a metal passageway that sprayed clean water from both sides, washing down the remains of the murky Liffey.

I tracked down my family crew and basked in the congrats. We agreed it was essential to go to a pub for some celebratory pints, and I noted that Mulligan's—the famous Mulligan's of Joycean renown—was just a short walk away on Poolbeg Street. The place was packed with swimmers, identifiable by their dark blue T-shirts, spilling out onto the sidewalk with their pints of chocolate-brown Guinness. Clearly, Mulligan's was the unofficial, post-Liffey gathering place. We squeezed through the throng to get our drinks and even managed to find a table. (Confession: not a fan of Guinness, so I celebrated with a red ale.)

Since then, I've swum in a lot of places in Ireland, and one of the truly signature spots is Kerin's Hole at White Strand Beach, outside the town of Miltown Malbay in County Clare. It's a natural pool at the base of a cliff, where whole families—some in wetsuits, some in "skins"—take the plunge, shrieking as they hit the water, paying no mind to the wind and cloudy weather. Some years ago, the locals decided the place needed safety improvements, so a new cliff access was built, funded by community donations. Stone steps and a very strongly anchored metal ladder that leads into the water. It was so popular I never found myself alone there, except once. It was at low tide, so low that the bottom of the ladder was dry. I descended, figuring all I had to do was let go at the bottom and splash in. Then it hit me—I wouldn't be able to reach even the bottom rung to pull myself out. I've since learned, through several trying situations, that planning how you're going to get out of the water is the most critical factor in this kind of swimming. Would the tide come in soon, raising the water level enough that I could hoist myself out? I had no idea. I don't live by the ocean, so I don't pay attention to this kind of thing. I could crawl out onto some slippery rocks, but that's another thing I've learned not to do when I'm alone. Reluctantly, I bailed. I went back up the ladder and walked five minutes back to the sand beach. I must be wiser in my old age.

In 2019, I flew solo to Ireland, and there was one thing that was non-negotiable: I determined to stay in places where I could get into the water. Every. Single. Day. Within a day of arriving in Dublin, I took myself to the fabled Forty Foot, a promontory on the southern tip of Dublin Bay where people have been plunging into the Irish Sea for centuries. It's not in the city of Dublin proper, but a mere 25-minute ride on the Dublin Area Rapid Transit system, known as the DART. There are various theories about how the Forty Foot got its name, but it doesn't have anything to do with the depth of the water. It's less than forty feet, but deep enough for the brave souls who dive from its highest rock. I opted for the safe way, down an old stone staircase with sturdy iron handrails. There are many of these stair-and-ladder setups across the seacoast because the Irish accommodate swimmers. They encourage swimming, they make it easy. In contrast to North America, with all its do-this-don't-do-that warnings, in Ireland they *want* people to go in the water.

At Forty Foot, an ancient sign near the entrance reads "Gentlemen's Bathing Place," but I see plenty of females of all ages in the water. It's a peculiarity of Irish swimming spots that for generations many of them were designated as men-only. Irish women, definitely no shrinking violets, tolerated being barred from open water for only so long. In July 1974, a group calling itself the Dublin City Women's Invasion Force liberated the Forty Foot, marching onto the promontory with placards reading, "Out from under and into the swim" and "We will fight them on the beaches." As the women plunged into the water, some of the men yelled nasty things at them, but they must have known their time was up.

A couple of years ago, the Forty Foot took the number one spot on a *New York Times* list of "The 10 Best Places to Swim in the World, According to Me," modestly compiled by singer Loudon Wainwright III (father of Rufus and Martha). As wonderful and as historic as it is, my own visit didn't fully tick the Forty Foot off my bucket list (to the extent that I have one). The water was "a bit on the cool side" as the Irish say, but far warmer than would greet the crowds at the annual Christmas Day dip. The Forty Foot is legendary as a year-round bathing spot with its own dedicated cohort of winter swimmers, which I resolved to join, a goal that had to be shelved because of pandemic restrictions.

For my next excursion, I got off the DART one stop earlier than usual to check out the beach at Sandycove. It's revered both as a swimming spot and for its famed Martello Tower. There's a string of squat stone towers all along the coast, south from Dublin. They were built in the early nineteenth century as defenses against an attack by Napoleon's army, which never materialized. The one at Sandycove is *the* Martello tower where Joyce stayed in 1904, and later immortalized in *Ulysses*. It now houses the James Joyce Museum, with displays of some of his books, personal items, and rooms as he described them in the opening chapters of the book. There's even a plaster death mask of Joyce. I wondered how a person is chosen to be immortalized in a death mask. How important do you have to be?

I didn't manage to get out of the city every day, so I was reduced to checking out pools, those chlorinated, concrete tubs I usually avoid like the plague. It was hot in Dublin, and I wondered whether there was a way to swim again in the Liffey. I knew that, a few weeks hence, the river would be full of people for the hundredth Liffey Swim; but aside from that event, swimming is officially disallowed in the river. I also had to admit that the sludge on the walls at low tide made the prospect unappealing.

Fortunately, I was won over by a public fitness facility named for Countess Markievicz, the great heroine of the 1916 Easter Rising. Born Constance Gore-Booth, she grew up in County Sligo and married a Polish Count in her twenties. After the 1916 rebellion was quelled, Countess Markievicz was sentenced to hang, along with Patrick Pearse, James Connolly, and the other leaders; but her sentence was commuted because she was a woman. (It's reassuring to know, in this age of MeToo, that a woman was once spared violence because of her gender.) She was later elected as a member of parliament for Dublin but never took her seat because she refused to swear an oath of allegiance to the British monarch.

For swimmers, the city of Galway is truly the Promised Land. I stayed in Salthill, a neighborhood with a string of beaches along what's known as the Prom, a 2-kilometer (1.2-mile) walkway along the shore that ends at the famed Blackrock Diving Tower. To be clear, I wasn't keen on diving into Galway Bay from a height of 25 to 30 feet (7.6 to 9 meters)—um, make that not keen at all. There was a time when I might have considered it but I'm at a point in life when I have no need of thrills. I watched one fellow walk to the edge more than a dozen times, trying to summon up the nerve, then back away from the brink. When a friend came up to lend encouragement, he still hesitated. Finally he shrugged off his friend's pep talk and walked back to the stairway having decided he just couldn't do it. Even then he had second thoughts. It seemed the humiliation of coming down without having taken the plunge was too great to bear. He suddenly turned, broke into a run, and flung himself over the edge to the cheers of his impatient spectators.

There's a daily constraint at Blackrock. Unlike the Forty Foot, where the water is always deep enough, there are times at Blackrock when the tide is too low to allow jumping. Several times, I watched the lifeguards bring out ropes to cordon off the stairway to the tower. I asked how they knew when to put up the barricade. Unlike in North America, where there'd be procedures and measurements and protocols, their guidelines were simple: "See the top of that long break in the wall there? When we see that, we just shut it down till the water comes up again."

Like many Irish bathing spots, Blackrock has an interesting history. In the summer of 1885, which was especially hot, a group of rogue Galwegians placed a springboard at the edge of the promontory so they could jump in and cool off. The owner of the property, a certain Colonel O'Hara, removed the board and proceeded to do everything he could to make life difficult for the swimmers. To be an enemy of swimmers is to be deeply un-Irish. Still, it took more than twenty years to resolve the matter. In 1910, the Urban Council managed to persuade the Colonel to lease a public right of way for £1 a year, and the rest is history. As in the battle against land enclosures in eighteenth-century Britain, the commons prevailed.

The present tower was built in 1954 and blessed by the parish priest of Salthill, who pronounced it "the finest diving tower in the country" (and no, it wasn't the only one). What's extraordinary about Blackrock is the culture that's developed around it. You want inclusive? There's old, young, male, female, slim, fat, and skin of all colors. They're all there, and not just to swim, but for the camaraderie, the conversation, the craic. (I had to use the word at least once in a piece about Ireland!) And if modesty is your hang-up, you're in for a bit of a shock. Everyone changes out in the open. To be a true citizen of Blackrock, you must master the art of stripping in and out of your swimsuit while minimizing exposure of your private areas. I studied the procedure carefully. It varies from person to person, but mainly involves large towels and very quick movements. Some people even have robes that they change underneath, making them look like a moving tent.

There's a wonderfully welcoming atmosphere at Blackrock. The regulars swim there every day, and after a few visits some began to recognize me and asked where I was from. When I told them most people in Toronto would find it too cold to swim there, they laughed heartily. As another woman arrived with her swimming gear, one of the regulars turned to her. "Hey, weren't you just here?"

"Yes," she admitted. She was back for another quick dip, her second in the past hour. "What can I do?" she shrugged. "It's an addiction, isn't it?" We all nodded. Yes, it is.

Kicking the ancient stone wall is a long-standing tradition as part of a walk along the Prom. If you walk the full 2 kilometers (1.2 miles) to the end, you must kick the wall before turning back. Why? For good luck? To scare the fairies? No one seems to know. The origin of the practice is lost in the mists of time, which somehow makes it even more imperative to honor it.

CHAPTER 9

The Great Lakes:
My home waters

"THERE'S NO PLACE like home." It applies to bodies of water, too. I've lived all my life on the Great Lakes, and Lake Ontario has been my 'hood for the past four decades. Toronto Island, where I live and swim, is part of the traditional territory of the Mississaugas of the Credit First Nation. The name Ontario is thought to be derived either from a Huron (Wyandot) word meaning "great lake," or from *skanadario*, a word in the Iroquoian family of languages, translated as "beautiful" or "shining waters." The dual-origin possibility is due to the fact that before European contact, the lake was a border between the Huron Nation and the Iroquois (now known as the Haudenosaunee) Confederacy. In the fifteenth century, the Haudenosaunee drove out the Huron from their territory and settled the northern shores of Lake Ontario. Later, the Mississaugas moved into the area and called the lake *Niigaani Gichigami* or "leading sea" in the Anishinaabemowin language. European colonizers retained the earlier name of Lake Ontario, which now prevails.

Lake Ontario is more than a lake, it's part of the vast system of five Great Lakes, the others being Lakes Superior, Erie, Huron, and Michigan. By measurement, Ontario is the smallest, but it has a larger volume of water than Lake Erie because it's deeper, with a maximum depth of 802 feet (244 meters). The total volume of water in Lake Ontario is 393 cubic miles (1,640 cubic kilometers), a 15-digit number you might as well not bother trying to comprehend. For some reason, listing statistics is considered a necessity when talking about the Great Lakes, so I'll continue in that vein: In size, Lake Ontario ranks thirteenth in the world. Its average depth is 283 feet (86 meters), and the length of its shoreline is 634 miles (1,020 kilometers). The last in the Great Lakes chain, Lake Ontario serves as the outlet to the Atlantic Ocean via the St. Lawrence River. There have been periodic campaigns to have the Great Lakes officially recognized a Natural Wonder of the World, but it hasn't passed muster in the company of Mount Everest and the Great Barrier Reef.

Swimming in a freshwater lake feels most natural to me. Tidal bodies of water are another thing entirely. Once, Alec and I were in the Moray area of Scotland so I could swim while he visited single malt distilleries. We were near a place called Lossiemouth (the name should have been a warning, not to mention the proximity to Loch Ness) and if the abundant signage about the possibility of dangerous rip currents wasn't enough to convince me to avoid the beach, the huge swells pounding onto the sand sealed the deal. The tidal pool curving around from the mouth of the river was appealing: calm, and just deep enough in the middle to actually swim. I headed down the sandy slope into the water and started swimming back toward the river with a nice, even stroke, thinking. *Wow, I really am becoming a stronger swimmer.*

When I turned to go back, I realized it wasn't my swimming skill at all: A strong tidal current had swept me down and was resisting my efforts to swim back. I'd played in swirling river pools and eddies before, but this one was different—a strong, steady force, under the deceptively calm surface of the water. It was like running on a treadmill, or swimming in one of those single-lane endless pools. I moved my arms and kicked my legs, but barely moved forward at all. I saw a rock ahead on the shore and tried to swim past it with little success. The only way I could propel through the water was to touch the bottom with my feet and push my body forward. I was in no danger, mind you. I was only a few feet from shore and could easily have walked out of the river onto the sand. No panic. Through the combination of arm strokes and leg propulsion, I gradually made my way back to my start point. But I was amazed by how much effort it took and came away with renewed respect for the sea and the power of its tides.

With a lake, I know what to expect. I know how to handle myself in Lake Ontario. At least, I like to think I do. Yet, I once managed to get myself in much the same predicament as during my Moray swim.

It was a wild day on Lake O, too rough to actually swim. Instead, I amused myself by body surfing in the big waves near the eastern end of Ward's Beach, imagining a passer-by saying, "Isn't that dangerous?" and me scoffing, "No, I do this all the time!" Thinking I know—no, *priding* myself that I know—just how far out I can safely go; how close I can be to the rocks without getting dashed against them by the waves; thinking I'll get out of the water after riding one more wave, a big one! I head toward the shore, get caught in the big one's undertow and find, to my amazement, that I was swept out into deeper water. The seawall was racing by me though, in truth, I was the one racing by it. I didn't panic. No, I knew how to handle myself in water, but I was still getting pulled along. I swung myself right into a niche between some big rocks, and finally found one I could grip.

I held on, managing to keep myself from being swept farther out, then started to make my way back to shore along the seawall, finding rocks here and there to grab onto. I was surprised—no *shocked*—by how difficult it was to pull myself through the swirling water. I started to worry, thinking, *If I lose my grip on this rock, I'll undo the progress I've made toward shore.* Finally I lurched to where I could stagger on to shore, grabbed my clothes from the sand and headed to a sheltered spot to change.

It was only as I was pulling down my suit that I noticed the streams of blood running down my legs, from my knees all the way to my feet. I'd gotten quite banged up pulling myself along the rocks, but in the cold water, I didn't feel a thing. Nothing serious, just cuts and scrapes—the bloody streaks made it look a lot worse than it was; but the reality finally began to penetrate my consciousness: *I could have been in trouble out there.* I thought I knew Lake O, but I didn't. As in Moray, I should have had more fear, more respect for the lake's power, especially in the cold. The winter lake is a different beast from the rest-of-the-year lake. It's not just colder, it's also bigger, meaner. I vowed from then on that I'd stay well away from the rocks in rough water. I'd learned my lesson: *Don't mess with a Great Lake.*

WATER FEARS

More than once I've been asked: "Aren't you afraid of what's down there?" No, I'm not. I can't really explain why. Like all phobias, aquaphobia is irrational, but it's a real condition that a significant number of people share. I don't belittle it, it's just that I find the very idea odd because nothing could be further from my own experience. I'm afraid of a lot of things, but water is not one of them. I've swum many times in dark-ish water where I couldn't see the bottom, but I just didn't think about what might be down there. Part of the reason may be that I've never experienced a serious water emergency or, worse, come close to drowning. I can totally understand why people who've had those experiences may have a crippling fear of entering the water. There are other factors, not so extreme, that shape one's feelings about water. In her memoir, *Swimming Studies*, Leanne Shapton acknowledges her own fear of swimming in open water, one she shares with many other competitive swimmers whose natural habitat is the pool. But the simple explanation for my lack of fear is that I'm a freshwater girl. Most of my swimming is done in lakes, not oceans that swarm with critters, big and small.

Recently, I read about an ocean swimmer who was ensnared in the tentacles of a lion's mane jellyfish. Now that *is* a terrifying thought! On a trip to Ireland a few years ago, we arrived late in the day at our rental house in West Clare. I was desperate to get into the water, but the beach was a bit far, so I went in at the end of our road. It was rocky and low tide, not deep enough to swim. So I just sat in the cool water for a few minutes, thinking, "Oh, look at all these funny, round blobs floating around me." I figured they were some kind of jellyfish and later learned they're called moon jellies, and they sting! They say animals react when they smell fear, so maybe it was good I was so clueless sitting among them. It made me wonder if maybe it would be better if I were at least a teeny bit aquaphobic.

I'm not entirely immune from fear of water, though. The events of 2017 showed me that. There were record high water levels in the Great Lakes that year, causing major flooding in the region, and Toronto Island was not spared. The Great Lakes cycle through high- and low-water years, but this was my first experience of flooding. It wasn't dramatic, more like a disaster in slow-motion, but that didn't make it any less threatening. I've lived on this island for the bulk of my adult life and I love being so close to the water, but in "the year of the flood," the water was too close for comfort.

End to end, Ward's Beach is about 300 meters (328 yards) long. Little more than halfway down, a wooden bench set back into the trees. Over the years, I got into the habit of using it as a base for my towel and clothes, especially when it provided some shelter from a cold wind. The friends of a man named Stephen had acquired it from the city of Toronto as a memorial after his death, and it bore a simple metal plaque with his name, his birth and death years, and the words, "From friends who miss him still." I didn't know anything about him but that he'd passed away in his forties. Occasionally, I wondered about him and his truncated life.

Over the years the shoreline shifted, but the overall distance from the water to the bench was about 15 or 20 feet (4.5 to 6 meters), and it stayed fairly consistent. That changed abruptly and dramatically in 2017. I continued to use Stephen's bench—I had to, there was so little dry sand to leave my stuff on—but, day by day, the water edged closer. At the height of the flood, it felt eerie to sit on the bench with the water mere inches from my toes. By the middle of May, the footings of two metal lifeguard stands were sitting in the water. Much of the western end of the beach had disappeared altogether, and the main path leading there was under a foot of water. There's no fighting water. It wins every time.

Though the flood seriously affected the lives of people who live and work on the island, it didn't have an impact on my swimming, and yet, it did. I found it unnerving to watch the lake level rise with each passing day, to see how quickly and easily it could swallow a patch of land. I thought I knew the lake, that I'd seen her in every guise imaginable, but this was new and unsettling. Ponds and rivulets continuously filled and shifted. That summer, I never swam very far out from the bench, sometimes because of the waves, but sometimes simply because…I was afraid. Of what, I have no idea.

It was during "the year of the flood" that my 365-day swim companion, the Log Ness Monster, died an ignominious death. I watched with dismay as our resident Nessie was gradually sucked under the sand by the unrelenting high water until it disappeared altogether. A day later, it mysteriously rose up on the sand again, but there was something missing: its head. At first I thought the high water had somehow "re-sculpted" the beach sand and moved the shoreline farther out, which of course makes no sense, nor did it account for the missing head. I was certain no human power could have dragged it, filled it with sand, and moved it out of the water. As I explored the mystery with other beachgoers, what had happened became clear, revealing anew the awe-inspiring power of water. The previous night there had been a huge storm with fierce, crashing waves that pulled Nessie out into the lake, then repeatedly tossed it back on the sand, pounding and crashing until the head broke off. I was happy to hear that, while walking her dog, a neighbor had found the head some distance away from the body. She carried it back to her house and notified Tyler, its creator, that it was sitting on her front porch if he wanted to try re-attaching it. For several days the body continued to sit on the sand, majestic in its headless-ness. Then, one day, I came down to the beach, and Nessie was gone. Vanished. It turned out that someone had reported the wreck to city's parks department, which deemed it a "hazard" and sent workers to remove it. The angry lake had done its work, and the parks workers had finished the job, returning the Log Ness Monster to the earth from whence it came.

Farewell, my winter friend.

CHAPTER 10

Swimming into Old Age:
Older, colder, healthier

83-year-old Nina Maksimova, a Russian grandmother and champion ice-swimmer from Perm
won the first prize in the 25- and 50-metre
freestyle at the World Winter Swimming
Championship 2020 in Slovenia, footage
filmed in Perm on Friday shows. The temperature of the water was a shivering +1 Celsius
(33 Fahrenheit), though the swimmer said she
doesn't feel cold…it was not the first time she
took part in the competition of the kind, as she
holds around 40 medals. "At first I was third,
then I got silver medal, now the first prize. The
older I get, the higher the awards are."

—RT News Network, February 15, 2020

I STILL HAVE some years to go before I catch up to Nina Maksimova.

Earlier in this book I said cold water was the greatest anti-aging potion ever discovered, but I should clarify that. It's not like those high-priced, anti-aging creams. You won't look anything like the sleek women in ads when you're wrapped in a big-tent change robe with dripping wet hair. I don't swim to extend my life, but I've often joked that I swim in cold water to cryogenically freeze my body. What cold-water swimming does is make your "golden years" better, healthier. More than that, it changes your outlook in a profound way. It certainly has mine, though trying to explain how would force me into dancing-about-architecture territory.

The other day, a young woman on Ward's Beach expressed her admiration as I emerged from a swim in 9 C (48 F) water. "You're going to live forever!" she exclaimed. I replied that I wasn't really interested in living forever, but that postponing the end was an appealing prospect. On Swimtonic, one of the many outdoor swimming blogs in the UK, a man in his late seventies titled his post "Managing My Decline," which I think sums up the approach of most of us aging swimmers. "The times go up and the distances go down. I have almost accepted that now," wrote Allan White, who nevertheless believes that many of us will "still be doing amazing things at 75." In the course of writing this book and learning so much about this phenomenon, I've come to the conclusion that we elders are the real outlaw swimmers.

SWIMMING IN YOUR OWN BACKYARD

Those of us who have access to wild water in our own backyards are doubly fortunate. Take Ira Gershenhorn, for example. A web developer in his late sixties, he regularly swims in the Hudson River near his apartment on the Upper West Side of Manhattan. Users of the nearby bike path sometimes do double-takes when they see a human in water long considered dirty and unsuitable for swimming. From time to time, he gets kidded by passers-by who call out "Hey, Kramer!"—a reference to the *Seinfeld* episode in which Kramer gets fed up with his overcrowded local pool and starts swimming in the East River on the other side of Manhattan. Gershenhorn takes the kidding in stride but is frustrated by the prevailing attitude toward swimming in the Hudson. "They still think of the river as being polluted, but it's getting cleaner all the time." City officials agree, though they stop short of advising the public that it's safe to swim in the river, what with the currents, boat traffic, and difficult access into the water. Like Les Ourcq Polaires of Paris, the few brave or foolhardy souls who river swim mostly are left alone by the authorities. A strong swimmer confident in his abilities, Gershenhorn admits he's driven largely by convenience. He can be in the water within minutes of stepping outside his apartment building. When he first moved to Manhattan, he frequented beaches in Brooklyn and Queens, then thought, "Why can't I just jump in the river?" He recalled, "So I started doing that, and it was much easier. You don't have to spend the whole day going back and forth to the beach."

On the opposite coast, adjacent to the US–Canada border, retired journalist Peter McMartin had the same idea. He took up winter swimming to relieve the lack of structured time, what he termed the "ennui" of the pandemic. Fortunately, he lives a block from the ocean in Tsawwassen, a Vancouver suburb, where he can walk to Boundary Bay from his house, decked out in nothing but swimming trunks, a flannel housecoat, and a pair of Crocs on his feet. "When I first started walking to the bay, I expected people passing me on the street to either laugh at me or ask me what in hell I was doing, or, more likely, call the police because I appeared to be either a dementia patient who has wandered away from his care home, or a flasher. But no one did." A quick look of puzzlement might appear on people's faces, then they'd look away, leaving Martin to his peculiar fashion choices. He chalks up the muted reactions to Canadian politeness.

And every day, near the middle of the North American continent, residents of Toronto's Beach neighborhood are treated to the sight of another winter swimmer in a bathrobe and swimsuit. Christopher Hope, an eighty-two-year-old windsurfing enthusiast, decided to go full-on immersion and he surfs all year long, regardless of the weather. His morning routine never varies: "I get out of bed, I make my bed, I get into my swimsuit, put on my swimming shoes, and walk down." Hope follows the advice of Mike Tipton and other cold-water experts: He limits himself to no more than ten minutes in the water and wears a watch to monitor his time. Many tout the health benefits of enduring the cold water, from helping with joint pain and inflammation to relieving fatigue. Hope doesn't subscribe to those theories. He finds it mitigated the monotony of pandemic life: "A lot of people are COVID-bound and have nothing to talk about. Every day I go in, I email some of my friends and tell them what it was like."

If you want evidence of elder swimming as a worldwide phenomenon, consider the regulars at the Sai Wan Swimming Shed in Hong Kong.

Victoria Harbour, on the western tip of Hong Kong Island, is one of the world's busiest ports. Every morning, against a backdrop teeming with ferries, cargo ships, and fishing boats, some daring elderly swimmers dive into the choppy waters. They are rarely put off their routine, not even by inclement weather or imminent typhoons. Lau Sam-lan, 74, has been swimming there daily for about thirty years, one of many regulars who have been doing it for decades. The Sai Wan Swimming Shed, which they use as their base, has basic changing rooms and showers, housed in corrugated iron-clad huts. It harks back to a time in the mid-twentieth century when there were many similar sheds dotted around the harbor, but with worsening pollution and the arrival of chlorinated public pools, they fell out of fashion. Sai Wan is the last one standing. There are around eighty members of what has become a close-knit community, with the youngest in their fifties. Lita Wong is sixty-two and has been swimming there for twenty-five years despite the fact that there are two shared pools at her apartment complex. She prefers salt water.

Earlier in this book, I mentioned the remarkable cold-water adaptation of Japan's ama pearl divers. Perhaps even more amazing is that these women keep diving into old age, some well into their nineties. So much for the belief that old age is a time of frailty and vulnerability. Though there are no statistics to prove it, most of the people who jump into cold water worldwide are likely elderly. Over the years, I've encountered people who find it hard to believe I'm not worried about cold water giving me a heart attack. I'm happy to report that there's science supporting the idea of elders in cold water. In an online seminar in 2020, cold-water expert Mike Tipton put to rest the whole idea of age as a risk factor. In fact, he believes that cold water is a "great way to age gracefully" and that overall health, rather than age, is a far more important consideration. In Tipton's view, anyone with the right combination of "fitness and fatness" is equipped to handle the challenges of cold-water swimming. (This calls to mind the words of my late mentor Klaus Rothfels on the advantages of having "padding.") The one caution Tipton emphasizes is that older adults who have been cold-water swimming longer may have developed a greater degree of cold habituation. It's one reason I follow his advice to pre-determine my time in the water: "Don't go by how you feel, if you feel okay."

If anything, new research into dementia gives elders an even greater incentive to go cold. In 2020, early findings indicated the presence of a cold-shock protein in the blood of regular winter swimmers at London's Parliament Hill Lido. This protein was shown to slow the onset of dementia and even repair some of the damage it caused in mice. Professor Giovanna Mallucci, who runs the UK Dementia Research Institute at the University of Cambridge, says the discovery could point researchers toward new drug treatments that may help keep dementia at bay.

Drugs? Sure, fine. But I'm looking forward to the day when cold-water immersion is the prescribed treatment.

CHAPTER 11

Caring for the Water:
The woman who walked the Great Lakes

LIKE MANY OPEN-WATER swimmers, I've tended to slough off worries about water pollution. It takes more than an elevated E. coli count to stop me from swimming. I'm addicted to my regular water fix and would rather take my chances. Speaking of E. coli, I used to think it was a non-issue in cold water. Turns out I was wrong—E. coli can survive freezing. Still, in all the years I've been plunging into Lake Ontario, I've never been sick from swimming, though I know there are people who have, or who believe they have. I don't mean to minimize those anxieties. In times past, lakes and rivers routinely were contaminated with human waste, especially near urban centers. In recent decades, environmental groups have pushed governments to improve water quality and make these bodies of water safe for swimming. The Foundation for Environmental Education, an international organization based in

Denmark, has been at the forefront of this effort with its Blue Flag certification of beaches.

When beachgoers say, "Look at the pollution," they're usually pointing to a film of organic matter that collects on the shoreline—yucky, but harmless. (And yes, I know a toxin such as blue-green algae is anything but harmless, and I'm deeply grateful that Lake Ontario has been free of it, so far.) But for wild swimmers, organic flotsam and jetsam comes with the territory. For the most part, real pollution is the stuff you *can't* see in the water: heavy metals; PCBs; and the latest scourge of the Great Lakes, microplastics. As for day-to-day water use, most Canadians are fortunate to have unfettered access to clean water for drinking and washing. We don't have to think about it. The water we need is always there. That's not true for people who live on First Nations reserves. A large number of Indigenous communities live under boil water advisories and have for many decades. It's an enduring stain on governments in Canada, and a major reason why Indigenous people are leading the way in the fight for clean water in this country.

STEWARDS VS. USERS

> The Great Lakes are about 20% of the world's fresh surface water and we have it right here in the backyard of the upper Midwest so it's an incredible resource. The main challenge is to make sure it stays clean that it stays available to everybody who lives here.
>
> —Joel Brammeier,
> president and CEO of the
> Alliance for the Great Lakes

This seems like an accurate and perfectly neutral statement about our relationship to water. In the larger sociopolitical context, water is commonly referred to as a "resource" that is "available" for human use. This isn't meant solely in the extractive sense, of which the most egregious example may be the drawing, bottling, and selling of water by companies like Nestlé. Water is necessary: We drink it, we bathe in it, we cook with it. We literally can't live without it.

More recently, the concept of "blue space" has been gaining in popularity, in which proximity to water is associated with a range of psychological benefits for humans. A number of studies have concluded that spending time in and around aquatic environments consistently leads to improvements in mood and reduction of stress. It's a version of the popular idea of the moment that being in nature—enjoying "green space," and "forest bathing"—boosts our mood, reduces our stress, and even awakens our spiritual emotions. Both "water-as-resource" and "blue space" are evidence-based concepts that are concerned with the fulfillment of human needs.

We think of water as something that exists entirely for our use, or as something to gaze upon, such as a lovely waterfront view. At the same time, we see it as something apart from us, even though well over half of the human body is water. One way to describe our relationship with water is as "I-It," employing the language used by the early twentieth-century philosopher Martin Buber. His work focused on the centrality of what he called "dialogical relationships" in human society, and he warned against the impulse to relate to others as objects, not us, completely separate from ourselves: You exist for me, to serve my needs, my interests. What Buber termed the "I-It" encounter is an accurate description of how modern, industrial society views the natural world. What if, in the spirit of Buber, we were to shift our perspective and see ourselves *in relationship* with water? What if we become stewards rather than just users? What if, to paraphrase JFK, we ask not what water can do for us, but what we can do for water? It may sound odd, but in the early twenty-first century, that's exactly what one remarkable woman said we should do. To drive her point home, she "walked the walk" in a way no one had done before.

A GREAT LAKES WALKABOUT

Like many who live in this remarkable bioregion, I've swum in all five of the Great Lakes. For some, it's almost a bucket list thing, and a few people have been crazy enough to do it in a single day—which is possible with some night swimming, a good supply of towels, and a lot of driving. Two groups of cold-water swimmers pulled it off in 2016 and 2019 and published accounts of their 24-hour feat on the Internet. Their aim was to raise awareness about water issues and have fun in the process. But these hardy souls have nothing on Josephine Mandamin. She didn't swim in the Great Lakes. In fact, she probably never went into the water much above her ankles.

Grandmother Josephine *walked* the Great Lakes, all 10,000 miles (more than 16,000 kilometers) of shoreline.

A respected Anishinaabe elder from the Wiikwemkoong First Nation on Manitoulin Island, Grandmother Josephine's journey began in the early 2000s when she heard another elder's prophecy: that by the year 2030, fresh water would be so scarce that it would "cost as much as gold." She felt a calling to become a water protector, to raise awareness about pollution and water scarcity. In 2003, she embarked on a walk around the shoreline of Lake Superior, a remarkable feat that took her more than a month to complete. In surface area, Lake Superior is the largest freshwater lake in the world, containing about twenty per cent of the earth's fresh water. In the ensuing years, Grandmother Josephine led a series of ceremonial water walks around each of the other Great Lakes. On each one she carried a copper pail filled with water, was accompanied by other women, and flanked by a small group of men carrying an eagle staff. She also led water walks along rivers and other bodies of water till, eventually, her total distance walked for the water tallied more than 25,000 kilometers. As a point of reference, in that time, Josephine Mandamin walked more than half the circumference of the Earth.

What's astonishing is not just that she completed these marathon walks, but that she took it upon herself to do this in the first place. She is sometimes described as an "activist for clean water," but that doesn't begin to describe her role or the extent of her influence. Grandmother Josephine should be celebrated as much as the elite athletes mentioned in this book. Unlike them, she doesn't speak of overcoming limits or conquering the elements. Her intentions lie elsewhere.

For a time, I found it hard to wrap my ahead around what she was doing. Walking *around* water is the opposite of what I do; and literally *carrying* water, what was that about? Where was the political action? Where were the demands, the slogans? It took me a while to clue in to the full meaning of carrying the water: taking care of it, bearing the weight of it, nurturing it. It's almost the reverse of the way most people—including me—think of water, as holding, carrying, nurturing us. The purpose is more than political, it's ceremonial, ritual, or religious, if you like. Grandmother Josephine believes that water is a living thing, that water is a miracle, that it is sacred. Her signature phrase is "Water is life." Not "water is necessary for life." Water *is* life.

Josephine Mandamin came to Toronto Island in the summer of 2016. Supporters in a canoe had accompanied her as she walked the city's waterfront, and they arrived at

Ward's Island first, while Josephine took the ferry. A crowd gathered on the beach, while I (of course) swam out to welcome the paddlers. We gathered around a ceremonial fire while she spoke about the need for water protection and taught us a water song in Anishinaabemowin composed by Doreen Day, another of the Walkers.

Nibi Gizaagi'igo / Gimiigwechiwenimigo / Gizhawenimigo
(Water, we love you / We thank you /
We respect you)

My most vivid memory of that day is the moment the skies opened and dumped a huge downpour on our heads. The fire kept going. Nobody moved. Nobody ran for shelter. Oddly enough, other than when I swim, I *hate* getting wet. My house was only a short distance away, but in the moment I had no thought of running to it. I think everyone in the crowd felt that being part of the ceremony was a privilege, and staying through the rain was a mark of honor and respect.

Josephine Mandamin received numerous kudos for her water protection work: recognition from the Native Women's Association of Canada; the Anishnaabek Lifetime Achievement Award; the Ontario Lieutenant Governor's Heritage Award; and the Governor General of Canada's Meritorious Service Decoration, in recognition of her contribution to Indigenous leadership and reconciliation. In 2012, Toronto's Second Story Press (also publisher of this book) published a children's story by Joanne Robertson about Josephine Mandamin called *The Water Walker*. The book has since been translated into Anishinaabemowin and French and has been published in several countries.

Because of her age and health concerns, Grandmother Josephine announced she would take her last walk in 2017, and she called on other water walkers to take up the copper vessel and carry on her work. Josephine's own great-niece, Autumn Peltier, is one of them. Canadians know her as the thirteen-year-old who famously confronted Prime Minister Justin Trudeau at an Assembly of First Nations gathering in Quebec, in 2017. Trudeau had not even come close to fulfilling his sweeping election promise to ensure access to clean drinking water for all First Nations communities in Canada. Peltier let him know it, saying, "I am very disappointed in the choices you've made." A documentary about her called *The Water Walker* premiered at the Toronto International Film Festival in 2020, followed by an online discussion with another young environmental activist, Greta Thunberg.

In the wake of Josephine Mandamin's death in 2019, her influence has grown into a truly global movement of Indigenous water protectors. As I write, in the summer of 2021, two major water walks are in progress in North America led by women Josephine mentored. The Saskatchewan River Walk, led by Tasha Beeds, started in June in the Rocky Mountains, and follows the river eastward to Lake Winnipeg in Manitoba. She is an Indigenous studies scholar of Plains Cree, Scottish-Métis, and Bahamian ancestry, and has taken part in many previous walks. The group of women she is leading come from various First Nations—Mohawk, Woodlands Cree, Ojibway—and they will cover more than 1,900 kilometers (almost 1,200 miles).

In the US, Sharon Day of the Bois Forte Ojibwe is leading a Nibi Walk (*nibi* means "water" in the Ojibwe language, Anishinaabemowin) along the path of the Enbridge Line 3 pipeline. In mid-July, the Nibi Walkers set off from the shores of Lake Superior in Wisconsin and will end at the Minnesota–North Dakota border. Line 3, currently under construction in northern Minnesota, will have the capacity to transport nearly a million barrels of crude oil a day from the Alberta tar sands. The proposed line, which runs through Indigenous treaty territories and valuable wetlands, has encountered stiff opposition from Indigenous communities and environmental groups.

This is only a bare outline of what's happening in this movement. Water walks are ceremonial undertakings framed by specific protocols in the Indigenous spiritual tradition. They are regarded as a form of prayer. One way for those of us who are not Indigenous to think of them is as analogous to a pilgrimage. Many religions have a tradition of pilgrimage or sacred walk. On the last weekend of July, thousands gather to climb Croagh Patrick, the mountain in County Mayo named for Ireland's Catholic patron saint. The Hajj pilgrimage to Mecca draws millions of Muslims from around the world every year. Some pilgrimages have become more secular, such as the Camino de Santiago de Compostela in Spain, which attracts thousands of hikers who are interested in a physical challenge and personal development. They all share certain characteristics: leaving behind the concerns of daily life to walk long distances; often involving fasting and other forms of hardship; and they have a deeper spiritual purpose. An element that particularly defines Indigenous water walks is the way they draw on the generosity of others, both from afar and in the communities they pass through en route. This web of support is equally important.

Clearly, the Nibi Walks have a political dimension, given the lack of drinkable water on Native reserves and the larger harm caused by centuries of colonialism; but they don't want to be identified as slogan-shouting, sign-carrying activists. As Sharon Day puts it, "We are not protestors. Our only audience is the water." Another important part of the walks is that they honor the spirits of the ancestors who walked the land before them. The Saskatchewan River Walk goes through Tasha Beeds' maternal ancestral territory along the body of water where she grew up. Nibi Walkers welcome the participation of non-Indigenous people, as long as they share the intent of the walk, follow the protocols laid down by the Indigenous leadership, and come in the right frame of mind. "The water requires calmness, patience, kindness, respect and humility. If you are trying to walk with ego the water will humble you. If you are carrying anger, the water will quiet you." The water walk movement is rooted in Indigenous history and spiritual traditions, but it embraces all people and the whole of planet Earth. They aim at something deeper than a list of

specific demands: a wholesale awareness about the impor-
tance of water and our responsibility to care for it. "We
walk," Sharon Day says, "to draw attention to the simple
fact that without water, none of us will exist."

In modern urban life, where water flows with a turn
of a tap, we have lost touch with that simple truth. It's in
our self-interest to take care of our water, but more than
that, it's a moral imperative. The Indigenous relationship
to the waters of the Earth, so much deeper than the white
European world view, is rooted in the "Seven Generations"
principle, the responsibility to consider the impact of
human action on the next seven generations. Indigenous
people take the long view, both backward to their ancestors
and forward to their descendants. Our job is to follow their
lead and learn from them.

I love and respect the Nibi Walkers and I'm part of that
large web of support that helps sustain them. But at this
point in my life, I don't see myself going on an actual water
walk.

I'd find it too hard to stay out of the water.

CHAPTER 12

Even the Coldest Water is Life

DURING "THE YEAR of the flood," many of my Toronto Island neighbors answered the call for volunteers to fill and stack sandbags to hold back the rising waters. Eager to prove I wasn't some useless old lady, I stepped up to help. Bad idea. I could handle shoveling sand into the bags, but as I bent down to pick up one that was overly full, I ignored my inner voice screaming, "Don't do it!" Immediately, I knew I'd injured my back, which meant weeks of painkillers and restricted movement.

This had a profound and unexpected effect on my swimming. I could barely do a single stroke without pain. Much worse, though, was the fact that I couldn't face going into water that was even slightly cold. It was like I'd lost the tolerance built up over so many years. Even though I normally hate the warm temperatures whirlpools are kept at, I started using the one at the Y. It seemed to help, along with some physio treatments, and gradually I was able to swim more than a few strokes at a time. After a few weeks, the lake was starting to get a bit warmer and I found I could tolerate going in again; but I'd been swimming in the Y pool and found I didn't have much energy for open-water swimming. Short swims were all I could do, all I *wanted* to do. I felt sluggish, lethargic. My lake swimming didn't invigorate me the way it used to.

The back injury, and turning seventy, ushered in a period of self-doubt. Cold water had never let me down before, but now I found it wasn't enough to ward off my depression. Winter and the ice buildup on Ward's Beach came early that year, so I had to stop going in the lake. Since my 365 year I'd managed to do at least some winter swimming, but not that year. Dutifully, I kept up with my pool swims and didn't care much about conquering. Anything.

THE CELEBRITY SWIMMER, UNDONE

August of 2018 saw the return of the Toronto Island Lake Swim, a race with three courses of 750 meters, 1.5 kilometers and 3.8 kilometers (almost a half-mile, 1 mile, and 2.4 miles). I'd been involved with the event since it began a few years earlier and it had built up an enthusiastic following, but the swim had been canceled the year before because of the flood. (You might be thinking, "Why? There's plenty of water!" Yes, but the city of Toronto canceled all island events that year. Even ferry travel was limited.) The organizers were bringing it back and they wanted to make a big—bad pun alert—splash. One of them, Steve Hulford, said they wanted to feature me as one of several "celebrity" swimmers because of my 365 swim. The idea made me anxious, particularly in my state of mind at the time. I do best when nobody's watching and there are no expectations. Still, I appreciated the gesture, and assured Steve I'd be there.

Something was off the day of the swim. I just didn't feel right. It was nothing I could put my finger on, except my stomach felt a bit queasy. I wasn't really sick. The forecast called for unsettled weather and I guiltily hoped the swim might be canceled again. I'd completed the 3.8 kilometer twice before, at the back of the pack, but I finished, no problem. I considered doing the 1.5 kilometer instead, but decided that would be a cop-out because 3.8 is more than twice as long. I wished there was something in between. But I had to show my grit!

It turned into an ordeal like nothing I'd ever experienced in the water. The lake started out choppy and got worse as the afternoon went on. I kept thinking I was okay until, suddenly, I wasn't. I had told myself I could bail early, at the end of the third round of the course, but even that turned out to be a gargantuan struggle. I didn't see how I could make it. The big white inflatable arch marking the end never seemed to be getting closer. I tried every trick I could think of—singing in my head, counting strokes to 100—but I was done. In fact, I was undone.

I started to vomit. I never vomit! One of the spotters came over in a kayak and asked how I was doing. I always say cheerily, "I'm good!" This time, I wasn't, and I knew I couldn't—shouldn't—pretend otherwise. I felt furious with myself, but all I wanted to do was get back on land. I hung onto the back of the kayak, still barfing my guts out, and let her tow me all the way to the finish. I emerged to the traditional line of cheers and congratulations from other swimmers, but I didn't want anyone to even *see* me. I was one of the last out of the water even though I had only swum a little over half the length. So much for showing my grit. For days afterwards I hardly swam at all. The sight of waves made me nauseous all over again. I felt empty, spent. I knew it was the feeling of *having to measure up* that did me in. But the pressure was coming from within me, not from outside.

In early 2019, something propelled me back to the Memphremagog Winter Swimming Festival in Vermont. It wasn't a need to prove anything or keep up with anyone else, but a vague desire to reconnect anew with cold water. There's great camaraderie among the swimmers, who cheer on and encourage one another, plus a lot of talk about overcoming obstacles and testing your limits. I'd participated twice, and each time managed to win a medal for LTIW (Longest-Time-in-the-Water), a kinder, gentler way of saying "slowest."

On the last day of the winter swim meet, I was slated to do my final event, the 100-meter (328-feet) freestyle.

I'd been fine on the previous swims, and didn't think this length would be particularly daunting; but looking at all these people standing around the pool, I felt a bit fragile: fast swimmers; long-distance swimmers; lane-mates racing against each other, slapping one another on the back after their swims. As I entered the water, I thought about Grandmother Josephine Mandamin, the Anishinaabe elder known as the water walker. I'd learned of her death just a few days before Alec and I left for Vermont. She'd walked all those miles to teach us to care for the water. She went the distance, and now I had to get through a puny hundred meters of really cold water. As I started my strokes, I repeated her phrase in my head: *Water is life. Water is life.*

I got through the first two laps okay, but by the third lap it was getting hard. As I turned to start the final lap, I couldn't feel my hands at all. I paused a moment. The swimmer in the lane beside me had already finished. I had already accepted the fact that I was on my way to another LTIW medal. I lifted my hands out of the water and wiggled my fingers. Alec thought it might be some kind of secret distress signal shared by open-water swimmers, but I was just trying to make sure my fingers were still there, then I knew that I could finish the last lap. And I did.

Dead last, yet again. But not dead. Not yet.

Even the coldest water is life.

AFTERWORD

My 365 Covid Year

MARCH 13, 2020, a Friday. I should have known something bad was coming. Not that the evidence wasn't all around me: on the web, on the TV news. I mentioned to some neighbors that Alec and I had planned to go out that night to a jazz concert at a bar downtown, and was taken aback when one responded, "You're not going *out*, are you?" The music was sublime, but I had to leave halfway through when I realized I'd left my wallet earlier at Eataly, a foodie emporium. Someone had picked it up off the counter where I'd left it, and used my credit card at a local pot shop. (More than a year later, I still hadn't managed to replace my driver's licence because it wasn't possible to do it online.) The next day I'd planned to go to an all-day Irish music session at another bar, but at midnight full-on lockdown and stay-home orders kicked in. There would be no St. Paddy's Day in 2020.

That was the start of my Covid-19 year.

Who could have imagined that daily life would be disrupted so profoundly, for so long? Well, for starters, the public health professionals who'd been warning about the possibility of a worldwide pandemic for decades. As I write, things are starting to look a bit brighter. There are effective vaccines. I've had one shot, waiting for my second, and have nothing to complain about. I'm much better off than a lot of folks in this pandemic.

This whole book is written from the perspective that cold-water swimming is something I do because it feels good. But heading into November 2020, the ninth month of Covid-19, on what felt like the grayest, dreariest of days (which it wasn't, of course, any more than all other Covid days), I watched my mood tailspin. I thought—hoped!—my cold-water swimming would help me sail through the pandemic. But I felt paralyzed by doubts and negative thoughts: Why bother trying to write this book at all? Who cares whether I ever finish it? Who was I to write a book about cold-water swimming, anyway? I didn't belong in the company of the champions, the go-beyond-your-limits types.

I had to do something. I knew I was staring into an abyss, one I thought I was done with. I took some of the steps I'd taken before—going back into therapy; checking in with my GP about medication—and some I hadn't, such as starting online Irish bouzouki lessons! I decided to set myself yet another challenge. My 365 swim had brought me a huge boost of self-esteem a few years earlier.

I resolved to do it again. It would, of course, be in Lake Ontario because I knew for sure I wouldn't be going anywhere in the coming months. And this time there'd be no going to the pool as a fallback. I was determined to get into the lake every day of the winter, no matter what.

December of 2020 was relatively mild. No problem to keep going. By the last week of January 2021, though, things were touch-and-go. Bitter cold had set in, and ice was forming on Ward's Beach. One day, I walked right into some floating sheets of ice. They were thin and I knew they'd break up easily, which they did, slashing through the flesh on my legs and releasing a swirl of blood into water. Fortunately, it was so cold I couldn't feel a thing!

In February, some glorious skating ice formed on the island's inland pond. Perfect skating ice is a gift of nature that demands to be enjoyed immediately because it's so transient, so for a couple of days I didn't get *in* the water and substituted time *on* the water instead. A week into the month, ferocious winds pummeled both sides of the Island and brought huge waves, as big as we see them out here. I went to my secret spot on the harbor side, hoping at least for a dunking, but there was already ice buildup, with the waves bringing in big hunks to add to the shelf. I couldn't get anywhere near the water. I laughed to myself, *Accept it, Kath. You've done your best, but no streak this winter.* I started back toward my house, then decided to head back to the main beach to witness and "commune" (go ahead, laugh, that's how I thought of it) with the waves. And indeed they were frighteningly big.

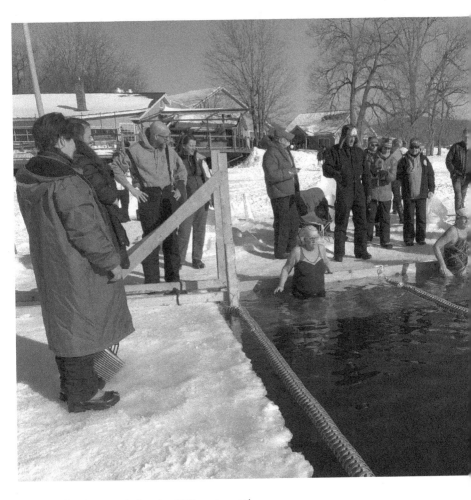

"Getting ready for the 100-meter at the
Winter Swim Festival in Vermont (2019)."
Photo by Alec Farquhar.

"Coming up to the finish line, Vermont (2019)."
Photo by Alec Farquhar.

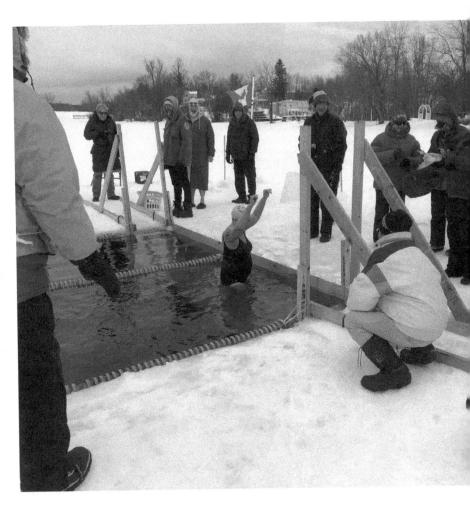

"'I still have hands!' Vermont (2019)."
Photo by Alec Farquhar.

There was no way I was about to venture in, but I noticed something else happening. The water level was still quite high from the second, lesser flood in 2019. Right on shore the waves were much smaller, gentler. A ridge of sand had formed from all the churning of the water, and after hitting it the waves ran out of steam (so to speak) several feet farther out from shore. As often happens on ocean beaches, ponds of sitting water had formed well back from the shoreline. They were only an inch or two deep (2 to 5 centimeters)—not much use for a dip—but near the rocks at the western end of the beach, one of the ponds kept refilling each time a big wave rolled in, creating a stream of swirling water that flowed in and out. All I had to do was strip down to my swimsuit, lie on the sand in wait for a good-sized one and—*pow!*—a nice, cold, exhilarating dunking! I was drenched, waiting for the next one—another *pow!* I threw on my jacket and pants and made my way back home where I discovered the waves had dumped more than water. There was a mess of sand inside my swimsuit. I showered it all down the drain.

It was totally worth it. I managed to keep my streak going right through the Covid-19 winter. As the pandemic wore on, it became clear that with the closing of public pools more and more swimmers were seeking open water than ever before. In my northerly neck of the woods, that meant *cold* open water. The boom brought a new burst of activity on and off social media. The Facebook group Swimming4Sanity started to help people deal with the isolation of the pandemic, and the anxiety and depression it brought with it. A member of another Facebook group urged fellow swimmers to conduct "citizen science" on themselves by wearing heart monitors and other devices to show that winter swimming could be done safely.

Across the country, there was a flood of TV news items, blog posts, and articles about people who were taking the plunge into cold water. One of them was mine. On New Year's Day, 2021, the *Toronto Star* ran a full-page feature with photos and the headline, "Toronto Island resident swims in Lake Ontario all winter and loves every freeezing minute of it." Here's part of what I wrote:

> There are countries like Russia, Iceland and Ireland where swimming year-round is fairly common. But when I first got into this odd pastime, I didn't have a whole lot of company. That has changed over the past decade, with the emergence of organizations like Britain's Outdoor Swimming Society and a growing number of Open Water swimming groups on Facebook. For the past few years, there's even been an annual Winter Swim Festival in Vermont, where organizers cut a 2-lane, 25-metre "pool" out of the ice in Lake Memphremagog, which straddles the border with Quebec. It's a strictly no-wetsuit event, and draws dozens of participants—strong, middle-aged swimmers of a somewhat, er, portly bearing. Because it's no surprise that certain bodies—ones with more

fat—are better equipped to handle the cold....
Sadly, the organizers recently announced that
the 2021 festival will, like all in-person events
these days, be cancelled.

(This turned out not to be true, strictly speaking. Like
everything else, the festival went virtual. And if anyone can
get a handle on the idea of virtual swimming, it's the folks
in Vermont.)

Yet, in the throes of this world-wide pandemic,
something remarkable is happening in the
swimming universe. Suddenly, everybody wants
to swim outside. In the cold! Since the early
days of Covid-19 lockdown, retailers of wetsuits
and other cold-water gear report big growth
in sales, and Facebook groups like Canadian
Cold Water Swimmers are seeing a surge of new
members. The phenomenon has spread across
the country, with groups who gather regularly
at Toronto's Cherry Beach, Okanagan Lake in
British Columbia, Halifax's Chocolate Lake,
even cutting ice holes in the Yukon. Quite a few
of these swimmers wear full wetsuits, while others (myself included) prefer to, in psychrolute
parlance, "go skins." Admittedly, there are other
ways to get your cold fix, like the followers of
Dutch "Iceman" Wim Hof, who post photos
of themselves sitting in chest freezers full of ice

cubes. But that's not my cup of (iced) tea; when
I'm in cold water I need to move.

The *Star* piece was followed by a bunch of radio interviews and an appearance on the satirical CBC show *This
Hour Has 22 Minutes*. They made fun of me, but in a nice
way. What I loved best was the stream of online responses
to my article and the gratitude they expressed. My cold-
water practice had long been a solitary undertaking, and
I was amazed that people felt so moved by it. Many were
purely congratulatory:

> *You're a brave person! I can't bear cold at all.*
> *I'm not sure I would have your stamina,*
> *but regardless, I'm envious of you.*

There was a few skeptics, though:

> *Good for you! But there's no mention of a buddy.*
> *Do you actually swim alone in cold water?*

(Damn—busted again!)

> *Thanks for the fantastic read. How do*
> *you manage not to suffer serious health*
> *issues that I have been taught about cold*
> *water? Exposure? Hypothermia? Shock?*

One reader told me about a group of women who swim every day of the year from a beach on the northwestern tip of Brittany. Another wrote about her friend who swims in the Ottawa River until it freezes over. Still another recommended a book called *The Finnish Way*, by Katja Pantzar, about the health benefits of going deep into nature, including swimming in the winter:

> *I've done several ice lake dips and have to say they're the highlight of my winter cottage-country excursions! It's exhilarating and meditative all at the same time. I highly recommend to anyone looking for an immune boost, mental rush, and natural high like no other! I'd certainly do this regularly if I had access to a body of water.*

Some recommended their own places for cold swimming:

> *My favourite spot to swim is Lake Superior which, even in summer is cccccooooooollllldddd. It is the most revitalizing, happy feeling I know. Every morning here in the city I try to recapture a few moments by ending each shower with pure cold Lake Ontario water. It is a way to wake up and feel alive, ready to face a new day with vigour! Like you, I am not a very good sportswoman, but this little ritual makes me feel like superwoman (for a few minutes anyway)! Thanks for the inspiration!*

A few unwittingly confirmed my observations on cold water and menopause:

> *I swim in Lake Ontario too. I started in my 50's because of a planter fasciitis issue. Needed exercise because I couldn't walk long distances. Realized quickly it managed my hot flashes and I sure got a healthy natural buzz from it. I have extra insulation that helps me deal with the cold but generally stay in for over a half hour. Use a suit in the off season. Everyone around me benefits from my happy water buzz. I use it for a meditation time and use the time for well wishes for others. It works for me so I totally relate to your article. Thanks for sharing. I think you are "cool" like me. Haha!*

As well as dogs....

> *I have an amazing Black Lab who doesn't hesitate to go into the lake this time of year if he's in the mood to. It's not for me, but now I have a better understanding of why others do it.*

I'm going to close this book with a couple of more lengthy replies. They moved me the most, probably because they were from people in the aging boat as I am. One was from a man in his late seventies:

I went back to the doctor: no football, no running, no swimming, no cycling; you name it and I can't do it. I disobeyed. Starting very slowly from a low base I rebuilt some fitness, better than average was the best I could hope for. And that is what I have achieved. I did lots of cycling and swam as often as possible, mostly in pools but lakes and sea during the holidays. I took up marathon running again. After these feats I suffered a natural slowdown, worsened by a series of injuries caused by adjusting for osteoarthritis, which ended in a total hip replacement. Running came to a complete stop. Crawl was just that, a crawl, but all I could do since breaststroke leg kick is known to dislocate new hips. Breaststroke gradually returned, but the weak kick on the mended side had to be matched on the good side to avoid swimming round in tight circles.

So, a mainly good physical life with two nasty setbacks taught me a valuable lesson, one that others have learned better than I did: You can only play your life with the cards that have been dealt. I find it hard to adjust and cope with having been a fair athlete and now having to deal with being among the slowest of the slow. It works if I focus on what I can actually do rather than regret what I can't do any more.

The other was from a woman around my own age:

> *The real gift for me is being able to swim year round.*
> *I've lived seaside for the better part of 40 years, and*
> *this is my first year swimming in the winter. But,*
> *I'm not alone, there has been a significant uptick*
> *in cold water swimming. I wish I had discovered*
> *this earlier. This is one of the best things to come*
> *out of Covid for me. I'm going to get serious for a*
> *moment. Covid has presented lots of challenges for*
> *my mental health, as I'm sure it has for most of us.*
> *I admit that I have an easy lot and my burden hasn't*
> *been onerous, but nevertheless I've felt like I was in*
> *a Covid fog and rudderless. Cold water swimming*
> *has lifted the fog and made this neverending Covid*
> *more manageable. In fact I welcome my morning*
> *cold shock and swim afterwards. It feels like a reset.*
>
> *It is amazing how a hit of icy water can wash*
> *away the darkness and lift the mood.*

To all that, I say a big Amen.

ACKNOWLEDGMENTS

I've enjoyed my time working on this book—both the swimming part and the writing part. As I say in the book, the former has been a fairly solitary activity, but with the latter, I've had a lot of help.

Several people read the manuscript at various stages. My spouse Alec Farquhar and my dear friend Annie Szamosi had very good things to say, and encouraged me to keep going. I'm grateful to Lynne Cox for her supportive, careful reading, which helped me avoid some errors and gave a real-world context to her astounding, trailblazing achievements. Dr. Heather Massey helped provide the book with a solid scientific grounding, based on her own research and cold-water experiences.

Like the best editors, Talin Vartanian was both supportive and demanding, to the book's benefit and mine.

My thanks also go to…

Kathryn Borczak, for sharing her thoughts about swimming an ice mile;

Donal Buckley for sharing his own ice mile and other cold water experiences;

Phil White, for letting me use that empty lane for an out of-competition lap;

Anne Barber for loaning out her copy of Waterlog for much longer than she anticipated;

Caitlin McDonnell, for being my swim buddy at Coney Island and various semi-frozen rivers;

The fabulous women at Second Story Press—Gillian Rodgerson, Melissa Kaita, Phuong Truong, Emma Rodgers, Bronte Germain, Jacqueline Downie, Michaela Stephen, and, of course, Margie Wolfe. And Bonnie Hewitt for her careful proofreading.

I'm grateful for Canada's commitment to its artists, and in particular for the support of the Ontario Arts Council and Artscape's Gibraltar Point Centre for the Arts while I worked on this book.

SOURCES AND RESOURCES

CHAPTER I

The recent swim memoirs mentioned in this chapter will be easy to find. But here are references for the ones that influenced me the most:

Haunts of the Black Masseur: The Swimmer as Hero, by Charles Sprawson. University of Minnesota Press, 1992.

Loneswimmer: The World's Best Guide to Cold and Open Water Swimming. www.loneswimmer.com

"The Swimmer," by John Cheever. Published in *The New Yorker*, July 18, 1964.

"Water Babies," by Oliver Sacks. Published in *The New Yorker*, May 26, 1997.

Waterlog: A Swimmer's Journey Through Britain, by Roger Deakins. Vintage Books, London and New York, 2000.

The "klutz" quote from Lynne Cox is from a January 26, 2021, webinar "An Evening with Extreme Swimmer and Author Lynne Cox," sponsored by the Cary Memorial Museum in Lexington, Massachusetts.

CHAPTER 2
The dramatic events of June 26, 1954, are recounted in "The Killer Seiche of 1954," a Flashback column by Stephan Benzkofer, Chicago *Tribune*, July 28, 2013.

The best place to start to learn about all things Toronto Island-related is this website, www.torontoisland.org, maintained by the Toronto Island Community Land Trust.

The Great Hudson River Swim was sponsored by NYCSwim, a pioneering organization that promoted open-water swims in New York for two decades. In 2016, NYCSwim shut down operations as well as their website.

CHAPTER 3
You can read more about Sir Lancelot Shadwell at the *Dictionary of National Biography*, 1885–1900/Shadwell, Lancelot. Vol. 51.

The Blobfish Café website is still on the web but there's no evidence that anything has been posted since 2015.

One of the earliest scientific treatises on cold water (with a very long title) is "Medical reports, on the effects of water, cold and warm, as a remedy in fever, and febrile diseases; whether applied to the surface of the body or used as a drink: with observations on the nature of fever; and on the effects of opium, alcohol, and inanition," by James Currie, 1797, available at *The Wellcome Collection*, a free online library.

The Water Cure in Chronic Disease, by James Manby Gully. London: John Churchill; Malvern: Henry Lamb, 1851.

Dr. Gordon Geisbrecht's (A.K.A. Professor Popsicle) website. www.coldwaterbootcamp.com

Rescuer Glenn Wallace's account of the incident is available at the *KPW Outdoors* website, posted October 13th, 2020.

CHAPTER 4

This isn't a footnote kind of book, and much of the research on cold water and the human body is fairly new and still evolving. Here are the main sources I consulted for this chapter:

"Cold water immersion: kill or cure?" by M.J. Tipton, N. Collier, H. Massey, J. Corbett, M. Harper in *Experimental Psychology*, August 23, 2017.

The webinar presented in January, 2021, featuring Mike Tipton and Heather Massey is available on *YouTube*: "Cold Water Swimming Webinar with Prof Mike Tipton & Dr Heather Massey."

The "Ice Series" of videos sponsored by the World Open Water Swimming Association (WOWSA): Episode #1 features Ram Barkai and Dr. Otto Thaning: "The ICE Series Episode #1: Heart and Hypothermia in The ICE with Ram Barkai and Dr. Otto Thaning."

Episode #2 features Barkai, Tipton and Massey: "The ICE Series Episode #2: The Unspoken Topic of Recovery with Mike Tipton & Heather Massey."

Other informative articles:
"Cold Water Swimming: Your Questions Answered," *Outdoor Swimmer*, January 13, 2020.

"The Science of Cold Water Adaptation: An Academic Adventure," *Oregon Lake Bagging*, October 25, 2020.

"Extreme Journeys with Jaimie Monahan," *Wowsa*, April 18th, 2020.

One of the best ways to learn about cold-water swimming is by connecting with groups of people who are out there *doing* it. The grandma of them all is the UK-based Outdoor Swimming Society (OSS).

There are far too many social media groups to list, but in my experience, the Canadian Cold Water Swimming Facebook group, hosted by two of Canada's "Ice Queens" is an excellent site that allows you to connect with other swimmers to ask questions, arrange meet-ups, and get supportive advice.

CHAPTER 5

"Treading Water: A simple comfort during a global pandemic," by Ian Brown, *Globe and Mail*, July 24, 2020.

"What I Miss Most Is Swimming," by Bonnie Tsui, *New York Times*, April 10, 2020.

"Neoprene and afterdrop: how to keep swimming outside this winter," by Amy Fleming, *The Guardian*, October 29, 2020.

"The Subversive Joy of Cold-Water Swimming," by Rebecca Meade, *The New Yorker*, January 27, 2020.

CHAPTER 7

There is no end of web pages about the achievements of Lynne Cox and Lewis Pugh, two world-famous athletes, so to get you started I'll point you in the direction of their personal websites: www.lewispugh.com; www.lynnecox.com.

Donal Buckley, AKA. *Loneswimmer,* has a thorough discussion of his ice mile experience on his blog. www.loneswimmer.com

You can read about the three women who broke Canada's ice mile "ceiling" on the website *Swim Diesel*: "Canada's Ice Queens." www.swim-diesel.com

Wim Hof also has an abundant presence on the web. His main website is "Wim Hof Method." www.wimhofmethod.com

"Wim Hof says he holds the key to a healthy life—but will anyone listen?" by Erik Hedegaard, *Rolling Stone*, November 3, 2017.

"Nuala Shares Moore About Cold Water Swimming," Steven Munatones, *Wowsa*, October 20, 2020.

CHAPTER 8
Big River Man, a documentary about Martin Strel's attempt to swim the Amazon. *Revolver Entertainment*, 2009.

Strel Swimming Adventures is the company run by Martin's son, Borut Strel.

"Paris plunge: daily queues after city opens cleaned-up canal to swimmers," by Angelique Chrisafis, *The Guardian*, July 22, 2017.

Information about the history of the Liffey Swim (formally known as the "Jones Engineering Dublin City

Liffey Swim") can be accessed at the *Ask About Ireland* website. www.askaboutireland.ie

Information about the Blackrock Diving Tower can be found at the website *This is Galway*. thisisgalway.ie

"The 10 Best Places to Swim in the World, According to Me," by Loudon Wainwright III, *New York Times*, August 19, 2017.

CHAPTER 9

Many online sources state that the name "Ontario" is Iroquoian in origin. This is because the Wendat language spoken by the Huron people, who lived on the lake's northern shore as far back as the 15th century, is part of the Iroquoian family of languages.

Swimming Studies, by Leanne Shapton. New York: Penguin, 2012.

CHAPTER 10

"83-year-old Russian grandma wins gold at World Winter Swimming Championship," on Ruptly, includes various elder swimmers' stories, as well as general articles on the positive effects of cold-water swimming for older people.

"Managing My Decline," by Alan White, *Swim and Tonic*, September, 2017.

"The Hudson Swimmer," by Corey Kilgannon, *New York Times*, July 11, 2018.

"Coming in from the Cold," by Pete McMartin, *Vancouver Sun*, December 27, 2020.

"82-year-old Toronto man takes a morning dip in Lake Ontario every day of the year," by Olivia Little, *BlogTO*.

"In Pictures: Elderly harbour-dippers at the 'Sai Wan swimming shed,'" *AFP*, June 11, 2017.

"Could an ice-cold swim be an antidote to depression and anxiety?" by Karin Olafson, *Globe and Mail*, June 16, 2019.

"Could cold water hold a clue to a dementia cure?" by Justin Rowlatt, BBC News, October 19, 2019.

"Women cold water swimming in Gower to help menopause," by Will Fyfe, BBC Wales News, February 8, 2019.

"What Can We Learn from Swimmers of a Certain Age?" by Bonnie Tsui, *New York Times*, June 22, 2020.

CHAPTER 11

The Alliance for the Great Lakes website. greatlakes.org

"Blue Spaces: why time spent near water is the secret of happiness," by Elle Hunt, *The Guardian*, November 3, 2019.

"5 Great Lakes in less than 24 hours," by Elodie Brunel, *Great Lakes Guide*, December 11, 2019.

There's an abundance of material on the Internet about Grandmother Josephine Mandamin, but the place to start learning about her and the Water Walk movement she helped create is at the *Mother Earth Water Walk* website. www.motherearthwaterwalker.com

"Tasha Beeds: survivor, scholar and water walker," by Lois Tuffin, *My Kawartha*, June 29, 2018.

"Water Walk will walk in prayer along the route of Line 3," *NibiWalk*, July 16, 2021.

ABOUT THE AUTHOR

KATHLEEN MCDONNELL grew up in Chicago, Illinois, the second youngest of nine siblings in an Irish Catholic family, and has lived in Canada all of her adult life. She is the author of nine books of non-fiction and YA fiction, and more than a dozen plays. As befits a passionate swimmer, McDonnell lives on an island where she and her life partner, Alec, raised their two daughters, Martha and Ivy.